THE
7 HABITS OF
HIGHLY
HEALTHY
WOMEN

Discover Your Divine Design for Healing, Vitality, and Wholeness

MIRIAM RIGAL SPENCER

Book Design & Production:
Columbus Publishing Lab
www.ColumbusPublishingLab.com

Disclaimer

This book is for educational and inspirational purposes only and does not substitute for professional medical advice. The author shares her personal experiences as a Certified Health and Life Coach and Certified Cellular Health Coach. Nothing herein is intended to diagnose, treat, cure, or prevent any disease. Always consult with your healthcare provider before making changes to your wellness routine.

Paperback ISBN: 979-8-90183-010-9
Ebook ISBN: 979-8-90183-019-2

Printed in the United States of America
1 3 5 7 9 10 8 6 4 2

TABLE OF CONTENTS

From My Heart
to Yours

This book was born from an urgency — a calling to remember, to heal, and to rise.

It is for the women seeking a higher way — who know we are not machines, but miracles. That the body is not broken, but brilliant. That we were never meant to merely survive this world, but to transform it.

But most of all, it is for my children and grandchildren — whose health, freedom, and future mean more to me than words can express. I want them to know the truth, remember who they are, and live in a world that values wholeness, peace, light, and love.

I wrote this because I believe in a new world — one that begins with healing from within. One breath, one truth, one healthy habit at a time.

It's an invitation to remember who you are and how your body was divinely designed to heal.

As you journey through these pages, you'll discover **seven simple habits** that restore balance at the cellular level and renew your strength from the inside out. My promise to you is this: If you lean into these habits with openness, you will find **greater hope, renewed vitality, and a deeper sense of wholeness.**

Whether you feel weary, stuck, or simply ready for more, these habits will show you that healing is not only possible — it's already written into your design.

Miriam

Why This Book Found You Now

I didn't set out to write a book. I set out to remember. To heal. To wake up. It began when my mother came to live with us, and I stepped into the sacred yet demanding role of caregiver. Her presence opened my eyes — not only to her needs, but to the cracks in a healthcare system I had always trusted. I began to see that much of our "modern health" isn't really health at all, but management of sickness. And as I cared for her, my own health began to suffer under the weight of stress, fatigue, and disconnection.

Then, when my husband's health crisis struck, everything changed. A dear friend introduced us to the science of redox signaling molecules — and through them, I witnessed the miraculous intelligence of the body in a way I had never seen before. Healing, I discovered, doesn't always come from outside of us. More often, it comes from awakening what God has already placed within us.

That discovery led me to **Dr. Gary L. Samuelson and his wife, Iris** — owners and co-founders of Cellular Health

Coaching LLC — whose groundbreaking work in cellular health uncovered a divine blueprint woven into every cell, a pattern we are all designed to follow. Immersing myself in his ten foundational laws, I questioned, lived, and prayed over them, gradually distilling their wisdom into seven habits that became instrumental in my own healing and in the lives of the women I support.

You are not broken. You are brilliant.

These are not just health practices. They are spiritual invitations. Gateways to remembering. Rhythms that restore us to our brilliance.

This book is for the woman who has tried everything, yet feels something is missing. For the one who is tired of the noise and ready to listen to her body again. For the one raising children in truth, not fear. And for the luminous, divine woman who still believes — as I do — that healing is possible.

Here you will not find fear, but freedom. Not shame, but sacred permission. A return to yourself, to God, and to the rhythms that were designed to keep you whole.

If these words find you, I believe it's because you are ready. Ready to slow down. To wake up. To breathe again. To rise again.

Come with me. Let us walk these seven habits together — and remember the divine design written within us all.

As you move through these pages, you'll find reflections and practices to help you embody each habit. For those who wish to journey more deeply, I created 7 Habits in 7 Weeks — a companion experience that brings these principles to life, one week at a time. You'll find details at the end of the book.

For the Children — And the Ones Yet to Come

This book is for the children of the world.
For the little ones who have not yet forgotten who they are.
For my grandchildren — and for yours.

May you grow up in a world that is cleaner, clearer, and kinder.

May you trust your body, listen to your spirit, and follow truth — not trends.

May you never be imprisoned by the matrix of misinformation, but instead live in freedom, wholeness, and light.

Some say this is a dream.

I say it is a remembering.

It begins with each of us — choosing to heal from the inside out.

Spirit.

Soul.

Body.

Let this be your invitation back to truth.

Back to peace.

Back to who you've always been.

PART ONE

Discovering Your Divine Design

How My Journey Led Me to Rediscover
God's Design for the Body.

CHAPTER 1

The Wake-Up Call:
When the Promises of Modern Health Fell Short

*"Our culture has sold women a bill of goods: that we are destined
to decline and decay. In truth, we are designed for lifelong vitality."*
—Christiane Northrup, M.D

I thought I was bringing my mother home. In truth, I was walking her into a system that would never truly care for her. When she came to live with us at age 80, I was hopeful. Grateful. I pictured slow Sunday dinners, deep conversations, and a sacred final chapter we would write together. My husband, gracious as ever, welcomed her without hesitation.

But what followed wasn't peace. It was chaos.

The First Cracks in the System

"We'll have to wait and see."

"It's probably just age."

"There's nothing else we can do. You'll just have to live with it."

If you've ever heard words like these, you know the chill they carry — the emptiness in your gut, the disbelief that someone in a white coat could speak so passively about the life you love.

These words are the slow death of hope. They're spoken not always as a last resort, but often as a default in a system that has lost its soul.

I didn't see it all at once.

It came in fragments — in real life, in real pain, in the quiet desperation of people I loved most.

And once I saw it, I couldn't unsee it.

My Mother's Story: An Unplanned Initiation

The day I arrived to help her move, I expected packed boxes… Mom was always ready on time!

What I did not expect was 16 orange bottles lined up neatly on her kitchen counter.

"Mom," I asked, startled, "what are all these?"

She answered dryly. "They're my medications."

Sixteen. Every day. Many of them for over 40 years. My heart broke for her in that moment — for the years she had carried this silent burden without a system that ever asked how she truly felt.

I wasn't a medical professional, but I knew something was wrong. Too many pills. Too many side effects. Too few questions. And worst of all — no healing. Just maintenance. Just survival.

One week after she moved in, she fainted in the front row of the church while my husband was preaching just a couple of feet away. With help from the congregation, we rushed her to the ER. That was the first of many visits.

I became her advocate — her eyes, ears, and voice. Every appointment, I asked questions. Every night, I researched drug labels and side effects. And what I discovered made me furious.

One doctor switched her to a new blood thinner. The label clearly warned: *Not recommended for patients over 80 due to risk of excessive bleeding.* When I questioned it, the nurse waved me off.

The next morning, my mother woke with a nosebleed — the first in her life. The office brushed it aside. Months later, I learned that same doctor was being paid to speak at pharmaceutical events promoting that very drug.

Not every doctor was like this. One cardiovascular surgeon refused a dangerous biopsy, saying, "I won't let her go through with it." He treated her, not just her chart.

But he was the exception.

For six years we lived in this cycle — appointments, ER visits, new prescriptions. Her kidneys quietly failed after decades of "treatment" that never healed. I cannot shake the belief that it wasn't her illness that took her, but the interventions meant to manage it.

Voices from the Shadows

"I became a full-time nurse with no training. One week I was helping my mom shop for groceries; the next, I was decoding medical charts and begging doctors to listen." — Cynthia, 58

"My mother didn't die of cancer. She died from the complications of the treatments. We were never offered a second opinion — just the next drug on the list." — Renee, 46

Their stories echoed mine. Different details. Same pattern: piecemeal care, reactive medicine, and a heartbreaking absence of true healing.

The Hidden Epidemic: Women as Caregivers

Nearly 60% of unpaid caregivers in the U.S. are women — and research shows that women who spend nine or more hours a week caring for a sick spouse are twice as likely to experience depression.

I became one of them.

The role reversal — daughter to caregiver — was an emotional tightrope. Some days I was her daughter. Other days, it felt like I was raising a strong-willed child.

Her health declined under the weight of pills, not despite them. And that's when the questions began.

I realized: To care for someone else, I had to care for myself. Self-care isn't selfish — it's survival. Rest isn't a reward — it's a requirement.

Nate's Story: The Second Blow

I thought the worst was behind me.

Then one night, I heard a crash. My husband, Nate, had collapsed. The ER ruled out heart attack and stroke, but the pain in his arms persisted.

A neurologist diagnosed carpal tunnel, peripheral neuropathy, permanent nerve damage — and handed him a prescription.

I recognized it instantly. It was the same drug that had stolen my mother's vitality. We refused.

"There's nothing else we can do," the doctor said flatly. "You'll just have to live with it."

Weeks later, after catching the flu, Nate was prescribed an antiviral and antibiotic. The pain in his arms worsened. I was in my office reading the label — *Not for patients with nerve damage* — when he appeared in the doorway, his face contorted in agony.

We had told the doctor everything. She had the full story. And yet, here we were again.

For nine months, Nate endured the pain. We prayed. We tried supplements, devices, creams. Some helped. None healed.

Until one day, an unexpected answer came.

But that's for another chapter.

The Awakening

This chapter isn't just about what went wrong. It's about what I began to see.

The system wasn't designed to heal.

It was designed to manage.

And I began to wonder:

If the system doesn't care about healing…then what does?

That question would change everything.

And if you are a woman in your sixties or beyond, you may know exactly what I mean. You've lived long enough to see the system work for some things — and fail for far too many others. You've watched friends disappear under a list of prescriptions, and maybe you've felt your own body whisper that something is off.

You've earned the right to question the narrative, and you have the wisdom to hear the answers when they come.

This stage of life isn't about settling — it's about reclaiming. And your story, like mine, is far from over.

As a wife, a daughter, and a woman in my own right — I was awakening. In that awakening, I found my voice.

This is the first step to becoming a Highly Healthy Woman.

Not just informed, but empowered.

Not just reactive, but resilient.

It's time to return to truth. To hope. To healing. To our divine design.

Later, I would discover something I had never heard of before — a missing link in cellular health that could restore communication in the body in ways I had once only prayed for. Had I known then what I know now about redox signaling, my mother might have had a better chance at living stronger, longer.

After reading this book, you will share this knowledge. And with that realization, this is where your journey begins.

3 Early Warning Signs the System Is Failing You

1. Your care feels fragmented.
Every specialist is focused on one body part or symptom, but no one looks at the whole picture — or asks about your quality of life.

2. New prescriptions replace questions.

If every side effect is met with another pill instead of a deeper investigation, you're not in a healing plan — you're in a management loop.

3. Your intuition says, "Something's not right."
If you feel dismissed, brushed off, or pressured into a treatment that doesn't make sense for you or your loved one, trust your inner alarm. Pause. Get another opinion.

Remember: You are the CEO of your own health. Your voice, your questions, and your boundaries matter — more than the comfort of the system you're navigating.

CHAPTER 2

The Awakening:
Seeing the Body with New Eyes

*"The truth is like a lion. You don't have to defend it.
Let it loose. It will defend itself."*

—*St. Augustine*

There is a moment in every awakening when the lights come on — and suddenly, you see everything differently. For me, it wasn't a single lightning bolt. It was a series of sparks. A series of failures by a system I had trusted. A series of whispers from my own body, my own spirit. And eventually, those sparks caught fire, revealing truths that pieced themselves together like a puzzle I could no longer ignore.

But here's the thing about awakening: it doesn't always feel beautiful at first. It can be disorienting, even lonely.

My awakening wasn't a lightning-bolt moment. It was slow, steady, and born out of love and necessity. As I cared for my mother — and later, my husband — I began to notice a troubling pattern. The doctors and the healthcare system often offered solutions that didn't make much sense to me. One of the first turning points came after the blood thinner medication that nearly harmed my mother.

Something inside me whispered: *This isn't the only way.*

That's when I began to question. To listen not just to medical advice, but to my own intuition. I realized I had to unlearn many of the things I had been taught, in order to relearn a way of healing that felt aligned with both wisdom and truth.

This was the beginning of my awakening — learning to trust what I knew deep down, and discovering that the body has a divine design for healing when we learn to honor it.

This awakening opened my eyes to a deeper truth: Our bodies are not broken machines in need of constant fixing — they are divinely designed systems, created with the ability to heal, renew, and restore when given the right support.

For women — especially those of us who have been the rock, the caregiver, the quiet glue holding a family together — awakening can feel like standing on unfamiliar ground. We've spent decades tending to others, raising children, caring for partners, shepherding aging parents, and leaning on the systems we were taught to trust. Then, without warning, we find we can't lean on them anymore.

We start to notice cracks other people walk past. We begin to hear the language of symptoms without root causes. We see people we love blindly following routines that are slowly eroding their vitality. And then comes the question that can't be stuffed back into silence:

What if what I've been told... isn't the full truth?

The Grief That Comes with Clarity

The first time you realize the modern medical system isn't built to restore health, a quiet kind of grief settles over you. It's not loud or public, but it changes you.

This was the same system that had wrapped my mother in prescriptions for decades, that told my husband to "just live with it," that offered pills and procedures but almost never asked the simplest question: *Why is this happening?*

Our healthcare model profits from pain. It is structured to manage illness, not resolve it. You are told you need more tests, more pills, more interventions — but rarely are you invited to explore the root cause. Once that truth settles in your bones, you cannot unknow it. But in the ashes of that grief, something else begins to stir — the memory of how we were actually designed.

Why Many Women Wake Up Later in Life

Looking back, I see I'm part of a growing wave — women in our fifties, sixties, seventies and beyond — who are done being quiet about the truth. We've lived long enough to recognize the patterns: the pills that didn't heal, the doctors who never asked a deeper question, the decades we pushed through fatigue as if it were a normal tax on womanhood.

But there comes a day when something in us refuses to keep accepting what doesn't align. We begin listening to our bodies instead of silencing them. We start seeking out integrative approaches, ancient practices, and the kind of medicine that treats a person's spirit as much as their symptoms. We remember that healing was never meant to be outsourced.

This awakening is not just physical. It is spiritual. It is generational. It is a reclamation.

The Lie We've Been Sold

We've been told our bodies are machines — prone to breaking, dependent on outside repairs. We've been told chronic illness is inevitable, that fatigue is normal, that menopause is the beginning of our decline.

None of this is true.

The truth is, your body is brilliant. Women's bodies, in particular, are miracles of design — capable of cycling, shifting, birthing, bleeding, nourishing, and renewing. We were designed for resilience. And when we stop interrupting that design, the body remembers how to heal.

The Divine Blueprint

There is a divine intelligence woven into every cell. Every organ system knows how to self-regulate. Every cell carries instructions for repair and renewal. Hormonal, neurological, digestive, immune — each system is orchestrated with breathtaking precision.

We were not designed to decay. We were designed to evolve. Healing is not only possible — it is the body's default when given the chance. But that chance begins with remembering who we are and how we were made.

Nate's Breaking Point

The awakening deepened for me when it became personal again — this time, with my husband. Nate is the strong, steady type. The man who doesn't complain. But I could see the pain in his body and the dimming of his spirit. He couldn't do the simplest things without wincing. I had already walked the caregiver's path once with my mother; now I found myself walking it again.

We tried everything — lotions, supplements, devices, advice from friends — each new effort carrying a flicker of hope that quickly died out. The frustration was maddening. Why wasn't anything helping?

Then, by what I believe was divine orchestration, a friend sent me an email about something called redox signaling molecules. I didn't fully understand the science at first, but my spirit recognized the truth in it.

We decided Nate would try it. He applied the gel three times in five minutes, then 10 minutes later, he found immediate relief. Three weeks later, his pain was gone. His energy returned. His eyes lit up again — and with them, the man I knew.

I've started using these redox molecules myself — they come in both gel and liquid form — not because I was in crisis, but because I wanted to see their effects firsthand. This was about reconnecting the signal between our cells and the divine blueprint already encoded inside us.

Redox was not hype. It was a reminder. A reminder that the body is already brilliant. That healing is less about adding and more about restoring. That what we need is often already within us, waiting to be activated.

For the Woman Who's Waking Up

If you're feeling that flicker inside — that quiet but relentless nudge telling you there's more — listen. You are not broken. You are not losing your mind. You are waking up.

If you are a woman in your sixties, you've likely been the keeper of your family's health stories. You've seen fads come and go, watched medicine change, and carried the weight of caring for others while keeping your own pain quiet.

But now? This is the season where you get to turn that wisdom inward. You have the resources, the insight, and the freedom to choose differently. And when you do, you're not just healing yourself — you're showing your children and grandchildren what it looks like to age in strength, clarity, and truth.

This is your permission to stop waiting for the system to save you…and start saving yourself. You're part of a new generation of women reclaiming their wisdom, refusing to be silenced, and daring to believe that health is our birthright.

You are asking better questions. You are challenging systems that profit from your pain. And you are remembering the truth: Your body holds intelligence, your spirit knows the way, and your healing is holy.

So please, don't ignore the whisper. Don't go back to sleep. Don't wait for permission. You are already walking toward your divine design.

Signature Takeaway: The 3 Layers of Awakening

1. Physical Awakening — The moment you begin listening to your body instead of silencing it. You notice patterns, side effects, and your own needs in a way you never did before.

2. Emotional Awakening — The shift from resignation to responsibility. You stop accepting "just aging" and start asking, "Why not better?"

3. Spiritual Awakening — The realization that healing is not just physical, but part of your divine design. You remember that your body and spirit were made to work together.

Awakening isn't always dramatic. Sometimes it's quiet, gradual, and born out of everyday choices and questions. My awakening began when I stopped ignoring that small inner voice and started listening to it. Yours may begin the same way — by paying attention to the whispers in your body, the nudges in your spirit, and the truth that feels too strong to ignore.

This is the moment everything changes. Once you awaken to the possibility that your body was designed for healing, vitality, and wholeness, you can never unsee it. And that's the very place where transformation begins.

Your awakening is not the end — it is the beginning. And the first step to reclaiming your divine design starts with the very thing you are doing right now: breathing.

In the next chapter, we step into the very first habit of a Highly Healthy Woman — the rhythm that anchors all the others.

It's the habit your grandmother's generation lived by, your body is still craving, and our modern world has almost forgotten. And once you reclaim it, you'll wonder how you ever lived without it.

CHAPTER 3

Discovering the Habits:
Where Science and God's Design Met

"The more I study science,
the more I believe in God."

—Albert Einstein

Before I share these seven habits with you, I need to tell you where they came from — and the man whose work helped me see the fingerprints of God in the smallest spaces of our design.

His name is **Dr. Gary L. Samuelson** — an atomic medical physicist whose research changed the way I understood the human body forever. He's the one who pioneered the stabilization of redox signaling molecules outside the body — a breakthrough many scientists thought was impossible. His work didn't just introduce me to a new frontier in cellular health; it gave me language for what my spirit had always known: that healing is both a science and a sacred act.

Dr. Samuelson teaches ten foundational laws for cellular health. I took those, sat with them, practiced them, wrestled with them — and slowly, through prayer, trial, and the lived experiences of my own healing journey, I distilled them into **seven**

habits that spoke most powerfully to the women I work with.

One of them — sunlight — isn't in his original ten. But it became so central in my own restoration that I couldn't leave it out. These seven are not a replacement for his model; they're my heart's offering, shaped by science, Spirit, and the lived reality of being a woman who has walked through sickness, caregiving, awakening, and into health again.

When Seven Habits Rose to the Surface

When Nate began to heal, I found myself replaying the days in my mind. What had changed? What had we shifted?

It wasn't just the molecules — though they were pivotal. It was the way we had begun to live. A slowing down. A listening. A returning to patterns that felt both ancient and strangely new.

In the quiet weeks after his recovery, I started noticing something: There were **seven things** we were doing, over and over. Small, simple, but powerful. They weren't trends. They weren't complicated. And they didn't cost a fortune.

They worked together like strands of a braid — science, Spirit, and daily life woven into something strong enough to hold us.

I began seeing the same patterns in the women I admired — women who were grounded, vibrant, and ageless in the ways that truly matter. They weren't chasing the latest health fad. They were rooted in steady rhythms that nourished them from the inside out.

These habits became the **7 Habits of Highly Healthy Women** and of course, they apply to men as well. They are not rules to master. They are invitations to remember.

Breath — The Forgotten Medicine

Breath is the first rhythm of life—and the one we most often overlook.

It is always present, quietly sustaining us, even when we are unaware of it. Yet as life becomes fuller and more demanding, we often lose our relationship with this most basic support. We breathe, but we do not always *receive* our breath.

Breath is more than oxygen. It is information. It signals safety or stress, calm or urgency, ease or resistance. With every inhale and exhale, the body is listening.

When breath is shallow, the body braces.

When breath is steady, the body softens.

This is why breath is foundational. It reminds the body that it is supported—and that healing begins not with force, but with presence.

And the quiet gift of breath is this: it requires nothing outside of you. It is available in every moment, waiting to be remembered.

Hydration — The River of Life

I pair hydration with breath because both bring flow. Without flow, there is stagnation; without stagnation, there is life.

Most of us live in a state of quiet dehydration — and I don't just mean physically. We run on empty emotionally and spiritually, too. But water is more than something to quench thirst. It is movement, memory, and cleansing.

When I began drinking structured, mineral-rich water consistently, it was as if my body exhaled in relief. My cravings softened. My skin began to glow again. My mind felt clearer. Water carries life into every cell — and when your cells are nourished, they remember how to function with ease.

Nutrition — Food as Frequency

We've been taught to treat food like math: calories in, calories out. But the body isn't a calculator. It's an orchestra.

Food carries information — vibrational codes — that tell your body how to respond. Whole, living foods speak the body's native language. Processed, chemical-laden foods are static and noise.

The day I began to see food as medicine rather than a moral issue was the day eating became an act of reverence instead of guilt. Every bite was either confusion or clarity. And clarity tasted like freedom.

Movement — Energy in Motion

I used to think movement meant exercise, and exercise meant punishment for what I ate. Now I see it as prayer in motion.

Movement is how we remind the body it is alive. It pumps lymph, carries oxygen, strengthens bones, and awakens joy. You don't need a gym membership to reclaim it — you need intention. Stretch while the tea steeps. Dance while the soup simmers. Walk in the fresh air and notice the way the world greets you.

Sleep — Divine Repair Mode

For years, I wore my exhaustion like a badge of honor. I thought rest was a luxury. Now I guard it like treasure.

Sleep is when your body turns inward to repair. Your brain detoxifies. Your hormones reset. Your immune system rebuilds. This is sacred work — and it only happens when we surrender to stillness.

The night I stopped pushing past midnight and began honoring my body's rhythms, I noticed something miraculous: I woke up with energy instead of resentment toward the day ahead.

Sunlight — God's Original Activation Code

Before there was life, there was light.

Sunlight is not just warm — it is instructive. It tells your body when to wake, when to rest, how to regulate hormones, how to lift your mood. It activates vitamin D and supports immune resilience.

When I began greeting the morning sun, my sleep improved. My mind cleared. My spirit felt steadier. I realized — light doesn't just shine on us; it speaks to us.

Redox — The Spark of Cellular Communication

This is where my worlds of science and Spirit meet.

Redox signaling molecules are already in you — tiny messengers that help your cells detect, repair, and renew. But stress, toxins, and age weaken the signal over time.

When Dr. Gary Samuelson discovered how to stabilize these molecules outside the body, he accomplished what many scientists thought was impossible. His breakthrough didn't create something new — it restored what was already written into our biology.

The first time I tried redox, I didn't know what to expect. But I remember noticing a lightness in my body, as if something deep inside had reconnected. It wasn't dramatic — it was subtle, like a switch being flipped back on. My spirit recognized it before my mind fully understood.

For me, redox is more than science. It is sacred. It doesn't override your body or force it into balance. It simply restores the conversation your cells were designed to have.

That's the difference. Healing doesn't come from the outside in. It comes from remembering.

Why the Habits Work Together

Each habit is powerful on its own — but when they come together, the body begins to hum again. You might start with one — breathing more deeply, drinking more water — and feel a shift. That shift creates momentum.

The body loves rhythm. It loves to be supported, not forced. These habits are not hard. They are home. And home is where healing begins.

Together, they form a language your body already knows — the language of Divine Design. Breath, hydration, nourishment, movement, rest, light, and cellular renewal are not new ideas. They are the original instructions, written into you from the beginning.

When we weave them back into our lives, especially as women in midlife and beyond, we don't just improve our health — we remember our wholeness. We remember that healing isn't a miracle to chase, but a rhythm to return to.

By now, you already know that wisdom doesn't come from quick fixes — it comes from lived experience. These habits are not for the woman looking for another trend she can abandon in a month. They are for you — the woman who is ready to reclaim rhythms that nourish your energy, protect your clarity, and help you live fully present for the people and passions you love.

You've earned the right to live in alignment with your Divine Design — and to do so without apology.

Takeaway: The 7 Habits in One Breath

Breathe like you are loved.
Drink like you are a river.
Eat like you are sacred.
Sleep like you are safe.
Move like you are alive.
Stand in the light like you belong there.
Restore your signal like your life depends on it — because it does.

In the next chapter, we begin with the first and most foundational habit: **Breath**. It was the rhythm that carried you into this world — and it is the rhythm that can carry you back into clarity, peace, and healing.

PART TWO

The 7 Habits of
Highly Healthy Women

How Your Body Heals by Divine Design

Breath of Life:
Energy & Renewal

*"Then the Lord God formed the man from the dust of the ground
and breathed into his nostrils the breath of life,
and the man became a living being."*

—*Genesis 2:7*

The first gift God ever gave you was breath.

It was there before you had words, before you had thoughts, before you even had a name. It was the rhythm that announced your arrival to the world and the signal that you were alive.

And yet, somewhere between that first cry and the chaos of adulthood, most of us forget how to use it. We shallow our breathing, rush through our days, and hold our breath without even realizing it — as if bracing against life itself.

I remember one evening, caught in the middle of an emotional storm, when my body was tight and my mind was racing. Without thinking, I closed my eyes, inhaled slowly, and let the air leave me like a prayer. In that moment, my shoulders dropped. My heart slowed. My body heard me whisper: *You are safe.*

Breath is not just oxygen. It is Spirit. It tells every cell you are alive, supported, and capable of healing. And the best part? You carry it with you everywhere.

From Breath to Biochemistry:
How Inhaled Oxygen Becomes Energy

Most of us think breathing is simply air moving in and out of our lungs — what science calls *external respiration.* In that space, oxygen crosses into our blood and carbon dioxide departs. But beneath that, in quiet mystery, another process is unfolding inside your cells.

This is *cellular respiration*: the miraculous alchemy in your mitochondria where oxygen meets glucose to create ATP (adenosine triphosphate) is the cell's main energy source. It stores energy and releases it to power everything your body's cells do — movement, repair, and growth. Picture it as the sacred spark behind every heartbeat, every hormone, every thought. Oxygen doesn't just nourish us. It powers us at the most intimate level.

When breath is shallow, that spark grows weak. Cells shift to backup, low-efficiency energy pathways — like flickering a flashlight in fading daylight. This shift ignites inflammation, reduces resilience, and accelerates aging. But when breathing is deep and rhythmic, mitochondria hum with energy. Your cells remember their intelligence.

Every inhale becomes a whispered invitation: *You are safe. You can restore now.*

Your outer breath fills your lungs.

Your inner breath fuels your cells.

One draws life in.

The other uses that life to keep you whole.

Women, Aging, & the Breath: Vitality Connection

For women over sixty, breath becomes even more essential. Hormonal shifts after menopause — especially the drop in estrogen and progesterone — subtly change breathing patterns, reduce lung elasticity, and influence how efficiently oxygen is delivered to cells.

This isn't just biology; it is wisdom whispering, *"It's time to breathe with greater intention."*

Mitochondria, already less efficient with age, feel the difference. Less oxygen means less energy, more fatigue, more inflammation. But here's the blessing: Intentional breathwork can reverse much of this pattern. When breath is honored deeply — slow, nasal, steady — it becomes cellular nourishment.

It doesn't just calm the mind. It reclaims your energy from the inside out. It restores clarity. It rebuilds trust in your body. And it helps women age with resilience instead of resignation.

Nitric Oxide: The Breath's Hidden Gift

There's another miracle tucked inside your breath. When you inhale slowly through your nose, your body produces nitric oxide — a molecule so powerful that scientists call it a master regulator. It improves circulation, relaxes blood vessels, strengthens immunity, and even acts as a redox signaling messenger, helping cells decide when to repair and when to defend.

This is why nasal breathing matters. It isn't just calming. It's chemistry for healing.

My Story:
The Night I Discovered My Breath Was Failing Me

I didn't fit the stereotype. I didn't snore or wake up gasping. But my breath was being interrupted just enough to keep my body in a low-grade state of alarm. That meant my lymphatic system wasn't fully cleaning house at night, my hormones were out of rhythm, and my cells weren't getting the oxygen they needed.

Those middle-of-the-night wake-ups? Not divine inspiration. They were my body fighting for air.

For years, I thought I was sleeping just fine. Sometimes I'd wake at 3 or 4 a.m. for no reason — but I brushed it off. Then one day, my dentist gently delivered news I never expected: I was grinding my teeth, I was tongue-tied and lip-tied, and I was living with a form of sleep apnea.

I was stunned. I didn't fit the picture of "someone with sleep apnea." But he explained just how serious even a mild case can be — interrupting oxygen flow, straining the heart, and accelerating aging in ways I couldn't see. Suddenly, the fatigue, the restless nights, the subtle stress all made sense.

Healing Without a Machine

I didn't want a CPAP. Instead, I chose a gentler path: myofunctional therapy — simple exercises to retrain the tongue, jaw, and throat. I began taping my mouth at night to encourage nasal breathing.

Slowly, my breath became steady again. I woke feeling rested, without that jolt of midnight adrenaline. My clarity returned. My energy lifted. And something deeper shifted — my nervous system began to trust again.

Breathing on Purpose

You don't need expensive equipment to reclaim your breath. You only need to remember it.

Here's one simple practice you can begin right now:

Box Breathing

1. Sit or lie somewhere quiet.

2. Place a hand on your heart.

3. Inhale through your nose for 4 counts.

4. Hold for 4 counts.

5. Exhale through your nose for 4 counts.

6. Hold for 4 counts.

7. Repeat 4 times.

As you breathe, imagine this rhythm as prayer:

- Inhale — God's breath filling your body.

- Hold — divine light saturating your cells.

- Exhale — releasing fear, tension, and anything that does not belong.

Breath as Liberation

Fast, shallow breathing keeps the body locked in survival mode. Slow, deep breathing is an invitation back into rest-and-repair. One accelerates aging. The other restores life.

If you've spent years caring for everyone else and forgetting yourself…

If you've been holding your breath without even realizing it…

If your chest feels tight and your spirit tired…

This is your permission to pause.

Close your eyes.

Inhale fully.

Hold gently.

Exhale completely.

Feel your shoulders drop.

Feel your mind grow quiet.

Feel your body whisper thank you.

Chapter 4 Takeaway

Breath is your built-in medicine.

It grounds you in the present.

It tells your cells you are safe.

It is the first gift you ever received — and the one you can reclaim at any moment.

So right now… place one hand on your heart, the other on your belly.

Breathe slowly.

You are still alive.

And as breath restores the flow of Spirit within you, water restores the flow of life through you. Together, they are the first steps in returning to your Divine Design.

CHAPTER 5

Hydration:
Living Water: Healing Flow

"Water is the mirror that has the ability to show us what we cannot see. It is the blueprint for our reality."

— *Dr. Masaru Emoto*

The Water That Listens

Water is not just a drink. It is a messenger. A carrier of frequency. A medium for miracles.

From the womb we were formed in — to the tears we cry, to the blood that flows through our veins — water is the element of life. It moves with grace, listens without resistance, and responds to vibration. It holds memory, emotion, and consciousness. It reflects back to us what we are, and what we believe.

More than 70% of the human body is made of water. Even more remarkably, water makes up over 99% of the molecules in our bodies by count — more than any other element. It flows within us, around us, and through every single cell. It is the sacred river of life within the body — and it must be treated as such.

For women, hydration is more than a physical necessity; it's a form of preservation. It keeps our joints supple, our skin luminous, our minds clear, and our moods steady. As we age, our body's water content naturally decreases — which makes conscious, intentional hydration one of the simplest yet most profound ways we can preserve our vitality and radiance.

Water Holds Memory: The Work of Dr. Masaru Emoto

Dr. Masaru Emoto, a Japanese researcher, changed the way the world sees water. In his groundbreaking work, he exposed water to words, music, and prayer — then flash-froze the molecules and photographed the resulting crystals.

What he discovered was stunning.

- Water exposed to loving, positive words formed beautiful, intricate crystalline structures — snowflake-like and symmetrical.

- Water exposed to angry or negative language formed chaotic, broken patterns.

- Water prayed over in meditation — regardless of religion — formed harmonious patterns of stunning design.

His conclusion? Water is alive to us. It mirrors consciousness. It hears us, feels us, and responds accordingly.

While some critics challenge Emoto's methods, his work awakened an intuitive truth many of us already sense: Water is vibrational. It carries intention. It reflects frequency. And since more than two-thirds of our bodies are water, our thoughts, words, and prayers inevitably ripple into our health.

So, what happens when we bless our water? When we speak

gratitude into the glass before we sip? When we whisper: *"Thank you. I love you. Heal me."*

We're not just being poetic. We're programming the structure of water at a molecular level — and sending those healing frequencies to every cell in our body.

> *"If you want to understand the universe, think in terms of energy, frequency, and vibration."*
>
> — *Nikola Tesla*

Water, Words, & Energy

Our bodies are about 70% water — and water listens. What we speak shapes the very medium of our being. If words can change water, imagine what they do to the human heart — and the hearts of others.

What This Means for You

It means that what you drink matters — but so does how you think.

You are made of water — nearly 60–70% of your body is this vibrational, living element. Your brain is about 80% water. Your blood is over 90%. Every cell, every organ, every function depends on hydration — and not just the quantity, but the quality.

Your water remembers your inner dialogue.

Your cells feel your frequency.

When you hydrate, you're not just feeding your body — you're imprinting your intentions into your cellular being.

A *Sacred Pause*

So, ask yourself gently: What is my water remembering today?

What words are you pouring into your cup, your body, your temple?

Are you hydrating with peace — or panic?

Are you drinking in truth — or fear?

In every sip, there is a chance to renew.

Natural Water and the Divine Design

In nature, water is never still for long. It spirals, dances, and flows in patterns that give it life. This movement creates molecular structures believed to enhance absorption, conductivity, and energy flow. You find natural water in fresh mountain springs, glacial melt, and the juices of raw fruits and vegetables.

Dr. Samuelson, one of my greatest mentors in cellular health, defines natural water as water that possesses the same balance of electrolytes, minerals, and biological materials found in a pure mountain stream. He considers this kind of water highly beneficial because it is absorbed almost instantly into the blood, helps lubricate joints and tissues, cleanses organs, and supports overall cellular hydration and function.

Natural water is enriched as it flows through layers of soil, rocks, and minerals — gathering magnesium, calcium, and potassium. These minerals are crucial for bone strength, muscle function, and a healthy nervous system. They also help water stay in the body longer, enhancing true cellular hydration.

Unlike flat, chemically treated tap water, natural water retains vibrancy and taste — encouraging us to drink more and hydrate deeply.

Dr. Samuelson's Simple Recipe for Natural Water

- 32 oz. clean, filtered (non-fluoridated) water

- A pinch of sea salt (for minerals & conductivity)

- 5–10 drops of fresh lime or lemon juice (for electrolytes & pH balance)

This isn't just hydration — it's an energetic infusion for your body and spirit.

How Electrolytic Water Travels to Your Bloodstream

When you drink electrolyte-enhanced water—such as natural water with a pinch of sea salt and a few drops of citrus—it's absorbed almost immediately through your gastrointestinal tract. The process unfolds primarily in the **small intestine**, where dietary fluids, along with secretions, enter in large volumes. Here, **electrolytes (especially sodium)** are actively absorbed, creating an osmotic gradient that passively draws water across the intestinal lining into the bloodstream. In fact, as much as **80–85% of ingested fluids are absorbed here**, with the remainder absorbed in the large intestine. The presence of electrolytes also enhances absorption efficiency by promoting ion-dependent water transport—so your body receives hydration more quickly and effectively.

The Hidden Signs of Dehydration

Most people don't realize they're living in a chronic state of low-level dehydration. You might not even feel thirsty, yet your body quietly sends signals: lingering fatigue, headaches, dry skin or lips, sluggish digestion, joint stiffness, poor focus, sugar cravings, even anxiety or irritability.

These are not random annoyances. They are your body whispering: *"Please, hydrate me."*

The Beauty of True Hydration

When your cells are properly hydrated with structured, mineral-rich water, the difference is unmistakable. Your thinking clears. Your mood steadies. Your skin glows. Your sleep deepens. Aches lessen. Immunity strengthens. And yes — your redox communication improves, helping your body repair and renew with ease.

Hydration doesn't just quench thirst. It restores harmony to the whole symphony of your being.

Hydration and Cellular Communication

At the deepest level, water is the lifeblood of your cells. It delivers nutrients, carries away toxins, supports mitochondrial energy, lubricates joints, and allows electrical impulses to flow between neurons.

But hydration isn't just about how much water you drink — it's about how well your body uses it. Without minerals like magnesium, sodium, and potassium, water can pass through you without deeply nourishing your tissues.

Water is also the conductor of redox signaling — the communication system that tells your cells when to repair, replicate, or rest. Without adequate hydration, it's like trying to hold a conversation over a bad phone line. Signals are missed, healing slows, inflammation rises.

Think of your body as a bustling city. Redox molecules are the messages that keep order. Water is the transportation system delivering them. Without enough water, the city slows, repairs lag, and chaos builds. But when hydration and redox work together, the city thrives.

For women over sixty, this becomes even more important. With less body water, weaker thirst signals, and age-related mitochondrial decline, hydration can make the difference between fatigue and vitality, between brain fog and clarity, between accelerated aging and graceful resilience.

Emotional Waters

Water doesn't just carry nutrients — it carries emotion. Our tears, our sweat, our very blood are rivers of feeling. Notice how your mouth goes dry in fear, or how dehydration sneaks in during times of anxiety. This is no coincidence.

For women especially, hydration can be an anchor during emotional storms. Drinking slowly and intentionally during grief, stress, or transition becomes a physical way to steady yourself when life feels turbulent.

When we allow our emotions to move — through tears, through sweat, through water — we restore the flow in both body and soul.

Blessing the Water You Drink

Before you drink, take a sacred pause. Hold your glass with both hands, close your eyes, and offer it a blessing. This is more than a sweet ritual. Science confirms that water's molecular structure shifts with intention.

As it enters your bloodstream and flows to every cell, it carries the frequency you've just given it.

For me, blessing my water has become a private conversation with God. It's a reminder that I'm not just hydrating my body — I'm ministering to it.

Resource Highlight: Environmental Working Group

I cannot close this chapter without drawing your attention to an organization vital to our health and future: the Environmental Working Group (EWG). This community of 30 million people has spent the past three decades protecting environmental health by pushing for higher industry standards.

One of their most eye-opening reports, *The State of American Drinking Water,* reveals the widespread contamination of tap water across the United States.

Visit www.ewg.org to learn practical steps for reducing exposure and safeguarding your health.

Final Reflections

Water is not just hydration. It is information, vibration, and life in motion. Every sip is an opportunity to bring your body into alignment with the design it was given.

When we remember this, we stop gulping water absentmindedly and start receiving it like a gift. We begin to flow more easily in our own lives — more nourished, more radiant, more whole.

Bless your water.

Bless yourself.

And let the river within you remember where it came from.

Bridge into Chapter 6

As women, we are made of rivers. Breath flows through us like invisible air, water courses through us as the river of life, and together they create the foundation of vitality. But breath and water alone are not enough.

The truth is: your cells are also listening to what you eat.

Every bite is information. Every meal is a message. Food carries not just calories, but codes — vibrational instructions that tell your body how to respond, how to repair, how to rise.

For too long, we've been taught to treat food as math: calories in, calories out. But the body is not a calculator. It is an orchestra. And food is either music or static.

This is where the next habit begins.

The next rhythm in your Divine Design.

The next invitation to align your life with healing.

If breath is Spirit and **water is flow,** then **food is frequency** — a daily communion with the intelligence of creation itself.

CHAPTER 6

Nutrition:
Nourishing the Divine Body

*"Let food be thy medicine
and medicine be thy food."*

— Hippocrates

The Divine Relationship Between Food and Healing

Food is not just fuel.

It is relationship.

It is creation.

It is sacred medicine.

It is how the earth speaks to your cells — how the sun, soil, and Spirit come together in every bite to offer healing, nourishment, and life. Every single thing you eat either supports healing or creates resistance to it.

We've separated eating from meaning, reducing food to numbers, macros, and calories. But you were never meant to "count your way to health." You were designed to experience food in full relationship — body, mind, soul, and cell. And above all, you were meant to eat with love.

Food is one of the most profound ways you interact with the

world: How you eat reflects how you live, what you eat reflects what you believe, and why you eat reveals what you need.

It's time to return to sacred eating — and sacred healing.

Food becomes medicine when it's infused with love, not just nutrients.

Micronutrients vs. Macronutrients — Rethinking the Plate

Forget the old food pyramid. Forget portion sizes.

As Dr. Gary Samuelson, Atomic Medical Physicist, teaches: Our bodies don't heal because of calories; they heal because of **micronutrients**.

Macronutrients — carbohydrates, fats, and proteins — provide energy and building blocks. But without the spark of **micronutrients** — the vitamins, minerals, enzymes, phytonutrients, antioxidants, and trace elements — that energy cannot be used effectively. Micronutrients may be required in tiny amounts, but they are essential for every repair and regulation process in the body. They activate enzymes, neutralize oxidative stress, support DNA repair, and keep the body's communication networks clear.

> *"Micronutrients are 'cell nutrients.' There are only about 40 different types of micronutrient molecules needed by our cells."*
> — *Dr. Gary Samuelson*

Dr. Samuelson recommends filling at least half your plate with micronutrient-rich foods. Imagine a meal that glows with life: deep greens like kale and spinach, the earthy crunch of broccoli and cauliflower, the fire-bright colors of carrots and peppers, the tang of sauerkraut or kimchi, the mineral gifts of seaweed, the vitality of sprouts and microgreens.

Each food carries a frequency — a message your body knows how to translate into healing.

> *"True nourishment begins with cellular conversation. Fill half your plate with living, colorful, micronutrient-rich foods — and let your body remember how to heal."*
>
> *— Dr. Gary Samuelson*

The Top Healing Nutrients

Certain nutrients are so essential, they deserve to be named:

Magnesium calms the nervous system and supports sleep. Zinc strengthens immunity and speeds tissue repair. Vitamin C builds collagen and detoxifies, while iron fuels oxygen delivery to every cell. Omega-3 fatty acids feed the brain and soothe inflammation. Folate repairs DNA. Selenium protects the thyroid. Potassium balances electrolytes. Iodine supports metabolism. Calcium fortifies bones and enables nerve signaling.

Each of these is found most abundantly in whole, living foods: leafy greens, nuts, seeds, legumes, sea vegetables, citrus, berries, and vibrant vegetables.

When you bless your food and fill your body with nutrients like these, you are not just eating — you are awakening your divine design.

Food as Cellular Communication

What you eat doesn't just fill your stomach — it speaks directly to your cells.

Certain plant compounds, like the sulforaphane in broccoli or the polyphenols in berries, awaken your mitochondria — the tiny powerhouses inside your cells — to create more clean energy and slow cellular aging. Fiber and fermented foods nourish your gut microbiome, the trillions of microbes that regulate immunity, inflammation, and even mood. These foods don't just feed you — they feed the life within you that keeps you whole.

Food also writes directly on your DNA through a process called **epigenetics**. This simply means your lifestyle choices can turn certain genes on or off. Food becomes a signal, telling your body which pathways to activate: repair, detoxification, resilience — or, if we're not careful, disease.

And when we choose foods rich in antioxidants, minerals, and living energy, we quiet the fires of chronic inflammation — the root of most modern disease — and allow the body to heal.

Amino Acids — The Builders of the Body

Amino acids are the "letters" your body uses to write protein "sentences" — creating structure, function, and repair. Of the twenty amino acids, nine are essential, meaning your body cannot make them on its own. These must come from food.

They are the builders and messengers of life. They repair tissues, make enzymes and hormones, fuel immunity, and even support neurotransmitters that regulate mood and thought. They also play a vital role in redox signaling and antioxidant defense.

Plants carry these amino acids in abundance. Lentils, quinoa, hemp seeds, nuts, beans, and leafy greens all offer pieces of the healing puzzle. Your body, in its wisdom, knows how to combine them. You don't need to eat animal protein to get "complete protein" — you need variety, color, and life.

My Story: A Shift Toward Compassionate Eating

For me, this truth unfolded slowly.

As my spiritual path deepened, I no longer desired meat the way I once did. Something in me whispered: *This isn't aligned anymore.* Each week I found myself reaching less for chicken or beef, and more for fruits, grains, leafy greens, living foods. It wasn't about following rules — it was about following resonance. And with every step, I felt more peace.

It began to weigh on me: the suffering of animals, the pain in the food chain, the disconnect between what we value and how we eat. A spiritual life honors life. Not just human life, but all life.

Although I'm not fully vegetarian yet, I know this path is part of my evolution. Each time I choose differently, I feel lighter, clearer, more aligned with my soul. I am no longer eating just to satisfy hunger — I am eating to honor the divine design of my body, my spirit, and this Earth.

The Frequency of Food

Food is not only chemistry — it is frequency. It carries the memory of the soil it grew in, the hands that prepared it, the way it was harvested, and the intention behind its creation.

Quantum physics confirms what ancient wisdom always knew: Everything is energy, and energy has frequency. The frequency of food influences the frequency of your body, shaping vitality, mood, cellular repair, and spiritual clarity.

Foods that grow close to the earth, ripen under the sun, and are eaten in their whole form — fresh fruits and vegetables, herbs, spices, nuts, seeds, whole grains, and fermented foods — carry higher frequencies. They are alive, and they support life.

Highly processed foods, on the other hand, often carry little life force. Chemical additives, refined sugar, artificial dyes, and heavily processed meats weigh down the body. These foods are difficult to recognize, harder to assimilate, and they drain more energy than they give.

When you eat consciously, you reconnect with remembrance.

Food, Love, and Relationship

Love is nourishment too. Meals shared with love digest differently than meals eaten alone, rushed, or distracted. When I sit at a table with someone I love, the food tastes better, the mood feels lighter, and my body receives more than calories — it receives connection.

Healing is relational. Just as loneliness weakens the immune system, love strengthens it. Every meal is relationship: with your body, with God, with others, with the Earth. Eating in harmony with your divine design restores something sacred that our fast-paced culture has forgotten.

Joy is medicine. Togetherness is medicine. Relationship is medicine.

Eat Real Food, Not Chemicals

Much of what lines grocery shelves is not truly food, but profit-driven products laced with preservatives, pesticides, dyes, and additives. Real food wears the colors of creation — the green of spinach, the gold of turmeric, the deep violet of blueberries.

Whenever possible, choose organic, especially for crops most vulnerable to pesticide contamination. The Environmental Working Group (EWG) publishes their Dirty Dozen and Clean Fifteen each year. Even choosing organic for just the top offenders can dramatically reduce your toxic load.

Visit www.ewg.org to stay informed.

Grow Your Own

If you've ever picked a tomato from your own vine or pulled lettuce from soil you touched, you know something shifts. You remember food is sacred. You remember you are a co-creator.

You don't need acres of land. A pot on your porch or even one basil plant on your windowsill can reconnect you to the divine rhythm of life.

The Sacred Act of Eating

Most of us were taught what to eat. Few of us were taught how.

Eating is not just biological — it is spiritual.

When you slow down, chew, and eat with gratitude, you allow your body to actually receive the nourishment it was designed for. Chewing well signals enzyme production, improves absorption, reduces bloating, and helps shift the nervous system into "rest and digest."

Sacred practice: Put your fork down between bites. Breathe. Receive.

Timing matters too. Traditional systems like Ayurveda teach that digestion is strongest at midday, making lunch your most supportive meal. Avoid eating late at night, and consider intuitive or gentle intermittent fasting to give your body space to repair. Above all, listen to your body's cues — it is wise.

Emotional Eating: Healing the Hunger Beneath the Hunger

We've all done it. A long day, a hard moment, an empty feeling — and suddenly we're reaching for food to soothe what feels unmet inside us.

Emotional eating is not weakness. It is human. But food can't fill an unmet need for rest, love, or connection. Instead of shame, we can meet these moments with curiosity: *"What am I really hungry for?"*

Sometimes it's comfort. Sometimes it's peace. Sometimes it's love.

For some women, gentle fasting windows — 12 to 16 hours — support repair, reduce inflammation, and activate **autophagy**, the body's cellular renewal system. But fasting should always be approached with care and self-compassion, never punishment.

The goal is not restriction — it is presence.

Nutrition for Women Over 60

This season of life is a crossroads. Hormonal shifts, slower metabolism, and reduced mitochondrial output can make it harder to sustain the energy and vitality you once took for granted. But food becomes even more powerful now — a daily tool for resilience.

Calcium, magnesium, and vitamin D are critical for bone strength. Zinc, selenium, and omega-3s bolster immunity and protect against inflammation. Plant proteins and amino acids preserve muscle mass and help regulate hormones. Colorful fruits and vegetables provide antioxidants that slow cellular aging and guard memory and cognition.

Hydration and redox balance weave into this picture too. Water carries nutrients into your cells, while redox molecules amplify the signals for repair. Together, they keep your inner communication clear.

At this stage, cravings may shift. Sweet comfort foods or stimulants may tempt you, but your body is actually calling for trace minerals, healthy fats, or deeper rest. Listening closely to those whispers allows you to nourish yourself with wisdom instead of willpower.

For women over sixty, food is not just medicine — it is preservation. It is a love letter to your future self.

Food, Joy, and Blessing

Healing through food is not about rules or restriction. It's about joy — laughter at the table, meals shared with love, food eaten as prayer.

- Your cells respond to joy.
- Digestion improves with laughter.
- Your body listens when you speak to it with love.

Closing Prayer of Gratitude

Before you read these words, take a slow, deep breath. Picture yourself at a table set with the colors, scents, and flavors of the earth. Imagine the women you love gathered there — passing bowls, sharing stories, laughing.

Let your body soften into that image, and from that place, let this prayer rise:

"Thank You for this meal, for the hands that prepared it, and the life that gave it. May it nourish my body, lift my spirit, and serve the purpose for which I am created."

Bridge into Chapter 7: Movement — Energy in Motion

Food is sacred medicine, but it was never meant to work alone. When you breathe deeply and drink living water, you prepare your body to receive nourishment. When you eat foods rich in light and love, you feed your cells what they most crave.

But there is another truth we cannot ignore:

Your body was never designed to stay still.

Every cell in you longs for motion — the rhythm of walking, the joy of dancing, the stretch of reaching, the flow of circulation carrying nutrients where they belong. Movement is how your body distributes the medicine of breath, water, and food. It is how you take the gifts of creation and send them pulsing through your bloodstream, your lymph, your very life force.

If breath is Spirit and water is flow and food is frequency, then movement is energy in motion. It is prayer expressed through the body. It is gratitude made visible.

In the next chapter, we'll remember what our ancestors knew long before gym memberships or fitness trackers — that movement is not punishment, but celebration. It is one of the purest ways to return to your divine design.

CHAPTER 7

Movement:
Grace Over Guilt

*"For in Him we live and move
and have our being."*

—*Acts 17:28*

This verse reminds us that every breath, every step, and every stretch is rooted in God's presence — our movement itself is a reflection of His life flowing through us.

We were not created to be still. We were created to flow — to rise and stretch, to dance and laugh, to move in harmony with the earth and sky. Movement is not just about fitness. It is frequency. It is medicine. It is mood. It is how we return to life after stillness has left us stagnant.

In a world that idolizes productivity and glorifies the grind, many of us have traded movement for mental overdrive. We sit at desks for hours, scroll our phones, and call it rest — but it's not. It's disconnection from the body. And the longer we stay there, the more we forget that movement isn't just physical — it's energetic. It's the way our cells communicate, our blood circulates, our lymphatic system drains, our fascia unwinds, and our energy opens.

Movement heals.

My Movement Story: Grace Over Guilt & Joy

I'll be the first to admit — I don't exercise every day. I love to work at my computer, read, research, learn, and create. I'm not someone who watches TV, so most of my day is spent sitting — and yes, I know that's not great for my body. I live in a cold climate, and during the winter months, I don't like being outside. So, the idea of walking regularly when it's freezing? Not happening.

My husband, now 73, is the definition of disciplined. When he makes a healthy choice — diet, workouts, all of it — he keeps it. He lifts weights at the gym three times a week and always invites me along. I go sometimes, but the gym isn't my cup of tea, and in winter I can disappear for weeks like a bat in a cave.

Here's what I've learned about myself: I crave variety and joy more than repetition. I don't love the gym, but I do love movement in community and play — yoga with my daughter, Zumba with others, free-dancing at home, and short trampoline breaks every hour to interrupt long stretches at my desk.

I discovered something magical in free-form dancing. There's something deeply healing about letting your body move without rules, without mirrors, without judgment. It's not about cardio or calorie-burn — it's about liberation. When I dance freely, I feel like I'm releasing energy that's been trapped in my body for too long. It's movement medicine for my soul.

More recently, I bought a small trampoline. Nothing fancy — but powerful. I set a timer and take short breaks to bounce, stretch, and move throughout the day. Just a few minutes here and there, and it shifts everything — my circulation, my clarity, my energy. It's simple, but it works. And more importantly, it works for me.

Those are the rhythms that keep me moving — classes when I want community, and playful micro-moves at home when I'm deep in work.

I've realized that movement isn't about a gym membership or a "no excuses" mentality. It's about listening to your body, honoring your season, and finding ways to move that match who you are and how you live.

So, if you're not a marathon runner or a morning yoga warrior, don't worry. You don't have to be anyone else. You just have to move — in the way that brings you life. And remember: even one step, one stretch, one bounce at a time…it all adds up.

Movement + Cellular Healing: How Motion Heals from the Inside Out

Every part of your body — down to the cellular level — depends on movement. Stillness has its sacred place in prayer, meditation, and rest. But prolonged stagnation invites decay. In Traditional Chinese Medicine, stagnation is the root of disease. Movement is how we bring chi — life-force — back into flow.

When you move, even gently:

- Oxygen delivery increases, fueling mitochondrial function — the energy factories in your cells.

- Nitric oxide production rises, dilating blood vessels, improving circulation, and enhancing redox signaling.

- Lymphatic flow is activated — and unlike blood, your lymph has no pump. Movement is its lifeline for clearing waste.

- Redox signaling is amplified, encouraging proper cell-to-cell communication, repair, and immune activation.

Think of it this way: Every step you take, every stretch you hold, every sway of your body is like unclogging a stream. Suddenly the water flows again, carrying nutrients, oxygen, and energy where they are needed most.

For women, especially in the years after menopause, movement plays a vital role in restoring balance. It supports bone density, steadies mood swings, keeps the pelvic floor strong, and even reduces hot flashes and brain fog. When your hormones shift, movement becomes not just exercise but a stabilizer — a rhythm that tells your body: "I am safe. I am alive. I am strong."

Inside the Cell: The Molecular Benefits of Movement

Science has begun to confirm what women have always known intuitively — when you move, you feel better. But here's why, at the cellular level:

1. Enhanced Mitochondrial Biogenesis — Movement signals your body to make more mitochondria, which means more clean energy, better detox, and slower aging.

2. Improved Redox Balance — Gentle oxidative stress from movement strengthens your natural defenses and resilience.

3. Autophagy Activation — Old, damaged cell parts are cleared away, making room for renewal.

4. Telomere Protection — Regular movement helps preserve the protective caps on your DNA, slowing cellular aging.

5. Epigenetic Expression — Lifestyle choices, like movement, can switch on genes for repair and immunity, while turning down genes linked to disease.

6. Myokine Release — Muscles release compounds that act like a natural pharmacy, lowering inflammation and boosting whole-body healing.

It's astonishing when you think about it: Your muscles aren't just for strength. They are a **healing organ.** Each time you move them, they release medicine into your bloodstream.

For women over 60, this means that even light resistance training or gentle yoga can trigger powerful internal healing cascades. Your body may not crave marathons, but it does crave rhythm, flow, and strength.

The Power of Free Movement & Dance

Among all forms of movement, one stands out for its emotional, neurological, and cellular benefits: **free-form dancing.**

You don't need choreography. You don't need a class. You don't even need to be "good." Just turn on a song that moves your spirit…and move.

When I let myself dance freely, without mirrors or rules, I feel something loosen inside. The stuck energy in my body begins to flow again. My laughter bubbles up, my heart opens, and my soul feels lighter. For me, it isn't about performance. It's about liberation.

Free dancing has been shown to:

- Regulate the nervous system

- Stimulate dopamine and endorphins (your "feel-good" chemistry)

- Enhance memory and cognition

- Improve balance and coordination

- Release trauma stored in fascia and muscle

And beyond all that…it simply makes you feel alive.

The Science + the Soul of Dance

Research confirms what ancient traditions always knew: Unstructured dance heals. A 2021 meta-analysis in *Frontiers in Psychology* found that free-form dance reduces depression and anxiety, improves cognitive function, and enhances emotional regulation.

Why? Because it activates multiple brain regions at once — the motor cortex, prefrontal cortex, and limbic system — creating new neural pathways, improving plasticity, and helping the brain let go of stress. In simpler words: Dance helps your brain rewrite its story.

That's why many women describe dancing as a spiritual experience. It isn't just movement — it's medicine for the mind, body, and soul. It is a return to the body as sanctuary, a place of wisdom and joy rather than judgment or shame.

When I see women over 60 swaying to music — whether it's with their grandchildren in the living room, in a Zumba class, or in the quiet privacy of their own kitchens — I see the divine spark alive in them. There is radiance in that freedom. There is healing in that joy.

Movement and Aging:
Supporting the Body Across Seasons of Life

As we age, the body begins to change. Muscle mass naturally declines — a process called **sarcopenia** — which can begin as early as our thirties if we're not intentional about movement. With it comes decreased strength, balance, and metabolism. Left unaddressed, this quiet loss can make even simple daily tasks feel harder — and yet, it doesn't have to be this way.

For women in their 50s, 60s, and beyond, movement is about more than weight loss or fitness goals — it's about preserving mobility, protecting bone strength, and keeping flexibility so daily life feels vibrant and free. Gentle strength training, stretching, and joyful motion aren't luxuries — they're investments in independence and vitality.

That's why resistance training — even with light weights, resistance bands, or simple bodyweight exercises — is so important. Movement doesn't just slow decline; it rebuilds strength, restores energy, and rewrites the story of aging.

Here's what regular movement helps preserve and protect:

- **Lean muscle mass** → keeping you strong and independent

- **Bone density** → protecting against osteoporosis and fractures

- **Metabolic health** → stabilizing blood sugar and preventing insulin resistance

- **Balance & stability** → reducing the risk of falls and frailty

For women especially, post-menopausal estrogen decline accelerates bone loss. But weight-bearing movement — walking, dancing, yoga, or light strength training — becomes one of the most powerful natural medicines to counteract that decline.

And here's the encouraging truth: It doesn't have to be complicated.

Even a 15-minute walk in one direction and 15 minutes back, five days a week, can transform how you feel. Pair that with two or three short strength sessions each week, and your body will respond with vitality.

Micro-Movements, Macro-Impact

Movement doesn't have to mean hour-long workouts. Even two minutes of intentional movement every 30 minutes — a stretch, a bounce, a walk to the mailbox — can drastically improve mitochondrial health and metabolism.

Your body doesn't need perfection. It needs rhythm. Small steps done consistently are what keep your cells young and your spirit bright.

So, whether it's a walk around the block, a dance in the

kitchen, or bouncing on a trampoline while your grandkids giggle nearby — **every movement is medicine.**

Movement as a Spiritual Practice

Movement isn't just for health. It's for wholeness.

Across cultures, movement has always been a sacred act:

- Indigenous peoples dance to honor the seasons, ancestors, and Spirit.

- Sufi mystics whirl in devotion, spinning themselves into union with the Divine.

- Yogis flow with breath, aligning body, mind, and Spirit.

To move your body is to remember you are still alive. To sway is to say: *I am still here.*

What if you moved your body not to punish it, but to honor it? Not as performance, but as praise?

Movement is prayer in motion. It is the way your body speaks when words fall short.

The Science of Stillness: What Happens When We Don't Move

The modern world rewards stillness — screens, commutes, endless scrolling. But sitting is now being called *"the new smoking."*

Sedentary lifestyles are linked to:

- Cardiovascular disease

- Type 2 diabetes

- Hormonal imbalances

- Cognitive decline

- Depression and anxiety

- Loss of bone density and muscle mass

Even 30 minutes of intentional movement a day can off-set these risks. But it's not just physical stagnation we battle. Emotional stagnation shows up when we don't allow our bodies to shake, sway, or release. Energy becomes trapped, and the body holds what the soul needed to let go of.

A Simple Start: The Healing Power of a 30-Minute Walk

If movement feels overwhelming, start here:

Walk for 15 minutes in one direction. Then turn around and walk back.

That's it. Just 30 minutes.

Do this five days a week and you'll:

- Lower your blood pressure

- Improve circulation and lymph flow

- Support redox signaling

- Increase oxygen uptake

- Calm your nervous system

Healing begins where motion returns.

Final Thoughts: Movement Is Medicine

Your body was made to move — not just to burn calories, but to activate energy, awaken your cells, and realign you with the rhythm of life itself.

Movement is how the body prays.

It's how the Spirit expresses.

It's how the cells stay young.

Before there were gyms or apps, there was movement. The body already knew how to sway, stretch, leap, and dance. Movement is part of our divine design.

I believe movement is sacred — not punishment, but praise. Not performance, but presence. Every step, every stretch, every sway whispers to your cells: *You are alive. You are healing. You are whole.*

Bridge to Chapter 8: Sleep — Divine Repair Mode

And then, when the moving is done…comes the stillness. The holy pause. The night when your body turns inward to repair, restore, and renew.

If movement is prayer in motion, sleep is surrender in silence. It is the divine reset where your cells repair, your mind clears, and your Spirit is renewed.

In the next chapter, we'll step into the rhythm of **rest** — and explore why sleep is not weakness, but wisdom.

CHAPTER 8

Sleep:
The Healing Power of Sleep

*"Come to me, all you who are weary and burdened,
and I will give you rest."*

— Matthew 11:28

The Gift We Keep Pushing Away

Before a baby eats, walks, or speaks…they sleep.

Sleep is primal, divine, essential — and yet, in our culture, it is often the first thing we sacrifice. We praise early risers and late-night hustlers. We glorify the go-go-go.

And we forget that healing doesn't happen in the hustle.

We were not designed to live in constant motion. We were created to live in cycles, rhythms, and seasons. And in the sacred stillness of sleep, the body remembers how to heal.

Sleep is not optional. It is the sacred reset button that returns us to balance.

The Sacred Science of Sleep

Sleep is a divine design — a rhythm woven into creation itself.

From the cycles of the moon to the migration of animals, everything on Earth honors a sacred rhythm of rest and renewal. We call this the *circadian rhythm* — a 24-hour internal clock that regulates sleep, hormones, digestion, and even emotional balance.

Our bodies are built to follow the light and dark — rising with the sun and resting with the moon. But modern life has turned our rhythms upside down. Screens, stress, and artificial light confuse our inner clock — and our bodies pay the price.

Modern science is finally catching up to what ancient traditions have always known: *Sleep is medicine.*

When you close your eyes and drift into sleep, a miracle begins. Your body switches from "doing" to "healing," from "fight or flight" to "repair and restore."

Here's what happens while you sleep:

- Cells repair damage caused by stress, toxins, and daily wear.

- The glymphatic system (the brain's detox network) flushes out waste.

- Hormones rebalance — melatonin, cortisol, insulin, leptin, ghrelin.

- Growth hormone is released — promoting healing and repair.

- The immune system recalibrates, strengthening defense.

Most of this happens in *deep sleep*, particularly between **10 p.m. and 2 a.m.** — the "golden healing window." If you're consistently awake during that time, your body misses critical phases of restoration, leaving behind inflammation, brain fog, and fatigue.

Women, Sleep, and the Season of Change

For women in midlife and beyond, sleep becomes even more vital — and often more elusive. Hormonal shifts in perimenopause and menopause bring night sweats, restless legs, and changes in melatonin production. Lower estrogen subtly affects bone density, cardiovascular health, and even memory — all of which are deeply supported by consistent, restorative sleep.

Lack of sleep is not just about tired mornings. It accelerates aging, weakens immunity, and scrambles hormone balance. For women over 60, restorative sleep is both prevention and restoration. It guards bones, hearts, and minds.

When you choose to honor rest, you're not being indulgent — you are actively protecting your resilience, your radiance, and your wholeness.

Why Sleep Deprivation Is So Dangerous

Even minor chronic sleep loss (under 6 hours a night) can lead to:

- Weakened immunity
- Anxiety and depression
- Weight gain and blood sugar issues
- Memory problems and brain fog
- Higher risk of heart disease and stroke
- Faster cellular aging

The body cannot repair what it doesn't have time to restore.

Sleep less, stress more. Stress more, sleep less. It's a vicious cycle — but one that can be broken when we reclaim the sacredness of rest.

Rest as a Spiritual Act

In nearly every spiritual tradition, rest is holy.

- In the Bible, God rested on the seventh day.

- In yoga, yoga Nidra is called "yogic sleep" for the soul.

- In Chinese medicine, night is the time of yin — restorative, feminine, receptive.

In dream states, we receive guidance. In deep sleep, the veil thins between physical and spiritual. Healing happens not just in the body, but in the soul.

Theta and delta brainwaves — the same states reached in prayer and meditation — arise in deep sleep. Perhaps this is why God whispers most clearly when the world is still.

My Confession on Sacred Sleep

Let me be honest. I teach about healing…and yet, I still wrestle with rest.

"It's 11:33 p.m. and I know I need to sleep. I teach this…and yet I resist. I don't like going to bed, and I don't like getting up."

Some nights I stay up creating or writing, even though I know better. I know that from the moment we fall asleep until midnight, the "cleaning crew" arrives — the lymphatic system, the glymphatic system, the hormones, the cells. I know this, and yet, I sometimes push past it.

But here's the part I hadn't shared until now: I also discovered that my breath was silently interrupting my healing. A diagnosis of mild sleep apnea stunned me — I didn't snore, I didn't gasp. And yet, my oxygen was being disrupted just enough to keep me in a shallow, restless state.

I didn't want a CPAP machine. Instead, I found something gentler — *myotape.* It doesn't cover the whole mouth, but gently surrounds the lips, encouraging nasal breathing through the night.

And something miraculous happened. I began to sleep through the night — deeply. For the first time in years, I began to dream again.

Dreams come in the **REM stage of sleep** — the final stage of the cycle, often just before waking. Without enough total sleep, the body never reaches it. Without REM, memory, creativity, and emotional healing suffer. But when I started dreaming again, I knew my body was finally reaching that sacred stage of restoration.

To dream again was to know that healing had returned.

Creating a Sacred Sleep Practice

We don't just fall asleep — we transition. And that transition can be sacred.

- Dim the lights by 9 p.m.

- Avoid screens an hour before bed.

- Journal, pray, or breathe slowly.

- Sip herbal tea or soak in warm water.

- Make your room a sanctuary — uncluttered, dark, and peaceful.

Treat your bed like a temple. Your body will respond.

Forgiveness, Sleep, and Cellular Cleansing

Forgiveness, like sleep, cleanses the body. Holding resentment fuels stress hormones. Releasing it lowers cortisol, calms the nervous system, and makes space for rest.

Dr. Dispenza — Doctor of Chiropractic (Life University), focuses on consciousness and self-healing through mind-body coherence. Dr. Leaf — Ph.D. in Communication Pathology/Cognitive Neuroscience (University of Pretoria), focuses on neuroplasticity and thought management. Dr. Joe Dispenza says holding old emotions is like storing their chemistry in your cells. Dr. Caroline Leaf confirms toxic thoughts create inflammation in the brain.

Sleep becomes the meeting place of emotional and physical cleansing. Forgiveness clears the soul while autophagy clears the cells.

A Prayer for Sacred Sleep

"Thank you, God, for the rhythm of rest.
As I lay down tonight, I release the need to carry it all.
Cleanse my body. Restore my cells. Calm my thoughts.
Fill my dreams with peace and possibility.

And awaken me renewed, reconnected, and ready for what comes next. Amen."

Takeaway: Sacred Rest for a Divine Body

Your body doesn't just rest when you sleep — it repairs, detoxes, and restores every cell according to a divine rhythm.

The hours before midnight are your most powerful healing window. And REM sleep — the dreaming stage — is proof you've given your body enough time to reach the deepest repair.

For women especially, sleep is sacred medicine. It guards your bones, protects your brain, and balances your emotions.

Sleep is prevention. Sleep is restoration. Sleep is your birthright.

So tonight, as you surrender, remember:

You are safe.

You are sacred.

You are being healed…even in your sleep.

Bridge to Chapter 9:
Sunlight — God's Original Activation Code

As night fades and the first light of morning touches the sky, the rhythm of creation continues. Just as sleep restores the body in stillness, sunlight awakens it to action.

The rising sun resets your circadian rhythm, signals your hormones, and calls your cells into alignment with the day. If sleep is the body's sacred reset, then light is its sacred activation.

In the next chapter, we step into the gift of sunlight — God's original code for life, health, and renewal. It is more than warmth. It is instruction. And when you learn to receive it, you will discover how light writes its healing message across every cell of your body.

CHAPTER 9

Sunlight:
Light is Life

"And God said, 'Let there be light,' and there was light.
And God saw that the light was good."

— Genesis 1:3

How Light Heals, Awakens, and Protects the Divine Body

From the very beginning, light was God's first creative act — the original frequency of life. It was not just illumination, but activation. Light awakened the earth, stirred the waters, and began the rhythm of days and seasons. It brought clarity, growth, warmth, and healing — all of which are still encoded into the sunlight that touches our skin today.

Somewhere along the way, though, we began to forget. We were taught to fear the very gift that was meant to sustain us. We smothered our bodies with chemicals, hid ourselves behind glass, and began to live like we were separate from the light that was always meant to heal us.

Sunlight is the oldest medicine, the purest energy, and perhaps the most misunderstood nutrient in our modern world. But we forgot that we are solar-powered beings — and that without light, we wither not just physically, but emotionally and spiritually too.

But what if the sun was never the enemy? What if it is separation from the sun — not its presence — that makes us sick?

My *Island Beginning*

I was never afraid of the sun.

I was born on a tropical island in the Caribbean, surrounded by turquoise water, golden sand, and skies so blue they seemed to hum. Every morning, the warmth of the sun poured over everything like a blessing. It was our clock, our calendar, our comfort.

Even when I later moved to the Midwest, the sun remained my compass — a part of me no winter could erase.

I'll confess, there was a time I tried to replace it. During one long northern winter, I experimented with tanning beds, desperate for the glow I missed. But after one overzealous season, my skin turned an unnatural shade of orange. When my father visited, he took one look at me, smiled gently, and said, "Don't do that anymore." He didn't have to convince me — I knew in my gut it wasn't right.

Years later, that same father would pass away from untreated, non-lethal skin cancer and other complications. He had the cancer removed but never followed up with the doctor. His death left a quiet imprint on me — a reminder that health is sacred, that light is sacred, and that we must learn the difference between life-giving sun and the things that truly harm us.

Now, I seek the real sun. I step outside often, allowing its warmth to touch my skin and spirit. And every time I do, I feel that deep remembering — not just of my childhood, but of the ancient, eternal relationship between light and life.

What the Sun Really Does in the Body

When sunlight touches your skin, something sacred happens. Beneath the surface, invisible alchemy begins. Molecules awaken, hormones shift, energy is created. The body remembers its design.

The most familiar gift of the sun is Vitamin D, often called the "sunshine vitamin," but in truth it acts more like a hormone — regulating over 2,000 genetic functions. Just a few minutes of sunlight on the skin can trigger this powerful cascade, strengthening bones, balancing hormones, stabilizing mood, and protecting against illness.

But the sun's story doesn't end there. Light is medicine for the mind. When morning rays reach your eyes — unfiltered by glass or sunglasses — they set your circadian rhythm, your internal clock. Your brain begins producing serotonin, the "happiness hormone," lifting mood, calming anxiety, and anchoring emotional resilience. Later, when the day turns dark, that serotonin is transformed into melatonin, guiding you into deep, healing sleep.

Even your skin carries memory of the light. Controlled, gentle exposure has been shown to calm inflammatory conditions like psoriasis and eczema. In some cases, it even speeds wound healing by stimulating nitric oxide and reducing local inflammation.

And deeper still, at the cellular level, light activates the mitochondria — the tiny power plants within your cells. Imagine thousands of microscopic suns inside you, sparked awake by the rays outside you. This is where energy is created, where vitality is restored. Without light, those inner suns grow dim. With light, they thrive.

The sun does not just warm the skin. It speaks to every system, every cell, every rhythm of your being.

The Case for Sunlight at a Glance

- **Longevity & Protection** — Moderate sun exposure is associated with *lower overall mortality* and reduced risk of cancer and heart disease. In a 20-year Swedish study, women who avoided sun had a 60% higher risk of all-cause mortality compared to those with regular exposure (midwesterndoctor.com).

- **Circulation & Cellular Energy** — Sunlight charges the body's internal water structure (H_3O_2 lattice), creating an electrical gradient that boosts blood flow, lymphatic drainage, and detox pathways (midwesterndoctor.com).

- **Mental & Hormonal Balance** — Morning sunlight regulates circadian rhythm, increases serotonin (daytime calm, happiness), and supports melatonin production for restful sleep. (https://www.health.harvard.edu/mind-and-mood/let-the-sunshine-in-a-natural-way-to-make-serotonin)

- **Ancient Healing Legacy** — Before antibiotics, sunlight was recognized as nature's broad-spectrum healer. Physicians like Niels Finsen and Auguste Rollier used heliotherapy to successfully treat tuberculosis, wounds,

and even influenza — long before the age of pharma-
ceuticals. (Sources: Nobel Prize Archives; Journal of the
Royal Society of Medicine, 2002.)

- **UVA vs. UVB** — UVA light penetrates more deeply,
  influencing collagen integrity and causing oxidative
  stress in excess. UVB, though capable of burning with
  overexposure, is essential — it activates Vitamin D
  synthesis, strengthens immunity, uplifts mood, and is
  correlated with lower rates of several chronic diseases.
  Sunlight is not only warmth — it is information,
  medicine, and alignment for the body's divine design.
  (Sources: Holick 2007; Hart 2016; Gilchrest 2013,
  NEJM; Journal of Investigative Dermatology.)

Sunlight at a Glance

- Vitamin D Production → 15–30 minutes of sunlight
  stimulates Vitamin D, vital for bones, immunity, hormones, and mood.

- Emotional Balance → Sunlight triggers serotonin, stabilizing mood and protecting against Seasonal Affective
  Disorder (SAD).

- Circadian Reset → Morning light anchors the body's
  internal clock, improving sleep and energy.

- Skin Healing → Gentle exposure can reduce psoriasis,
  eczema, and even speed wound healing.

- Cellular Energy → Light "charges" your mitochondria, boosting vitality and immune strength.

Your body is not simply warmed by light. It is informed by it.

The Sun and Cancer: Rethinking the Fear

Somewhere along the way, we were taught to fear the sun. To cover ourselves, to hide from it, to slather our skin with chemicals that promised safety. We were told that sunlight is the enemy — that every ray carried danger.

The modern fear of sunlight can be traced to decades of campaigns that cast ultraviolet exposure only as a danger, largely driven by dermatologic convention and industry reinforcement (Juzeniene & Moan, 2012; Norval et al., 2020). Yet data from a 20-year Swedish cohort revealed that women who avoided the sun faced a 60 percent higher risk of all-cause mortality than those who embraced moderate exposure (Lindqvist et al., 2014).

But when I began to look deeper, I realized the truth is far more nuanced.

Not all skin cancers are the same. The most common forms — basal cell and squamous cell carcinomas — rarely spread and are often easily treated. Melanoma, the most serious type, has been linked not to daily, steady sunlight but to something very different: intense, intermittent sunburns, often in those who spend most of their lives indoors.

The real story is that moderate, consistent sun exposure may actually protect us, not harm us. Research has shown that women who avoided the sun had higher mortality rates than those who embraced it. Other studies have linked sunlight exposure to lower risks of breast, colon, and prostate cancers. In fact, populations who live in sun-rich equatorial regions often have lower rates of melanoma than those in northern, industrialized nations who spend their days inside.

One study from the 1940s compared two groups of animals exposed to the same amount of UV light. Those fed a poor, nutrient-deficient diet developed skin cancer. Those fed a nutrient-rich diet did not. The conclusion was stunning: sunlight itself was not the villain — it was the internal terrain of the body that determined its response to light.

And isn't that what we've been learning all along? That health isn't just about avoiding risk, but about strengthening resilience. That when the body is nourished, balanced, and aligned with its design, the very things we were told to fear may become allies.

So perhaps it's time to stop vilifying the sun — and instead to ask a better question: What inside of us needs healing so that light can do what it was always meant to do?

Sunlight & Cancer at a Glance

- Basal Cell Carcinoma → Most common, rarely spreads.

- Squamous Cell Carcinoma → Low mortality, often treatable.

- Melanoma → The most serious; linked more to intermittent, intense burns than steady daily sun.

Research Highlights

- A Swedish study of 30,000 women found that those who avoided the sun had higher mortality rates than those who embraced it.

- Populations in sun-rich equatorial regions often have lower melanoma rates than indoor-dwelling populations in northern nations.

- A 1940s animal study revealed that poor diet, not sunlight alone, triggered skin cancer under UV exposure.

The takeaway: The real danger may not be the sun itself — but poor nutrition, chemical toxins, and lifestyles disconnected from nature's rhythms.

The Healing Spectrum of Light

Light isn't one color, but a spectrum of frequencies:

- UVB: The "Vitamin D light" — critical for immunity, bone health, and over 2,000 genetic functions.

- UVA: Deeper-penetrating; can be harmful in excess, but also helps release nitric oxide, which supports circulation.

- Red and Near-Infrared: Present at sunrise and sunset; reduce inflammation, activate mitochondria, and reset circadian rhythm.

That's why stepping outside in the morning is so powerful. The first light of the day — rich in red and infrared — calms the nervous system, syncs your inner clock, and whispers to your cells: It's time to heal.

Sunscreen: Friend or Foe?

Protection from overexposure is wise, but many commercial sunscreens contain chemicals that disrupt hormones and even create free radicals when exposed to light.

Safer choices include mineral sunscreens with non-nano zinc oxide or titanium dioxide, or using shade, hats, and clothing as natural protection. The simplest solution of all? Common sense: Avoid burning, but don't avoid the sun.

Bonus: Sunlight Enhances Cognitive Health

Studies suggest that sunlight exposure improves learning and memory — especially when paired with study or spiritual practices in the morning. Light influences brain-derived neurotrophic factor (BDNF), a protein that supports learning and neuroplasticity.

Light and the Feminine Body

Women's health is especially tied to light.

- Morning sunlight influences the hypothalamus — the master hormone regulator — supporting estrogen, progesterone, and cortisol balance.

- Adequate Vitamin D protects bones, strengthens immunity, and balances mood.

- For women in menopause, daily sun exposure becomes not optional, but essential.

We are not only nourished by food — we are nourished by light.

The Heart–Sun Connection

Indigenous traditions have long honored the rising sun as sacred. In Traditional Chinese Medicine, the sun is linked to the Heart — the seat of consciousness and joy and emotional intelligence. The Heart governs blood circulation, emotional balance, and the Shen (or spirit). Morning light is said to awaken the Heart meridian, fostering clarity and compassion. Imbalance in the Heart can lead to anxiety, insomnia, or restlessness.

I believe this is why, when I stand with my face to the rising sun, I feel both rooted and renewed.

Try this: Each morning, step outside within 30 minutes of waking. Let your eyes and skin receive the light. Breathe deeply. Whisper gratitude. Let your cells eat light.

Sunlight and Cellular Health: In Simple Terms

When you spend time in the sun, here's what's happening inside you:

- Your body makes Vitamin D — strengthening bones, immunity, and mood.

- Your circadian rhythm resets — helping you sleep, detox, and repair.

- Your mitochondria are activated — fueling energy and resilience.

- Your hormones find balance — supporting vitality, especially for women.

Sunlight is not just warmth. It is information for your cells.

Final Reflection: Let There Be Light in You

If you take nothing else from this chapter, remember this: The sun is not your enemy. Separation from it is.

When you align your body with natural rhythms — sun by day, moon by night — your cells remember how to heal. Light doesn't just warm the skin. It awakens the spirit. It informs the cells. It calls the body back into balance.

I have felt it myself — on cold Midwestern mornings when I finally stepped outside to greet the dawn. The warmth on my skin was more than comfort; it was medicine. It reminded me of my island beginnings, when the sun was our compass and our constant companion. And each time I turn toward it now, I hear the whisper again: You were made for the light.

So let there be light in your food.

Let there be light in your thoughts.

Let there be light in your cells.

Let there be light in you.

Invitation: Tomorrow morning, when the first light breaks,

step outside. Lift your face to the sun. Breathe deeply. Whisper gratitude. And let your body remember what it has always known: You are solar-powered, divinely designed to thrive in the light.

Bridge to Chapter 10: Redox

Sunlight doesn't just shine on us — it activates us. Every ray carries signals that spark communication at the cellular level, reminding the body of its divine design. And this brings us to the seventh and most revolutionary habit: Redox — the spark of cellular communication itself.

Because if light is life…then redox is the very language life speaks.

CHAPTER 10

Redox:
The God Molecule

"Redox signaling molecules are the fundamental messengers that allow cells to detect damage, initiate repair, and maintain health."

— Dr. Gary Samuelson

The Missing Link Between Cellular Repair, Energy, and Divine Intelligence: The Whisper Inside the Cell

There are moments when the body knows before the mind does — when fatigue, pain, or brain fog arrives without a neat diagnosis, only a sense that something deep inside has gone quiet. For my husband and me, that silence came as exhaustion and unexplainable pain. We searched. We researched. We prayed. Then one day, a dear friend called with something I had never heard of before — **redox signaling molecules**.

I was skeptical. It sounded too scientific, maybe too good to be true. But what began as a phone call became a divine redirection — the moment that introduced me to what I now call **the God Molecule**.

What Is Redox?

Redox is short for "reduction–oxidation," a foundational process in every living cell. It is the spark of life — an exchange of electrons that allows cells to sense damage, signal for repair, eliminate threats, and stay in constant conversation with the rest of the body.

Every second, trillions of conversations take place inside you. Cells repairing DNA. Immune cells coordinating defenses. Tissues deciding whether to rest, replicate, or regenerate.

Redox signaling molecules are the messengers. Without them, the conversation falters. And when communication breaks down, the body begins to lose balance. Inflammation rises. Fatigue deepens. Healing slows. Aging accelerates.

This is why redox is not just science — it is sacred.

Why Supplement If My Body Already Makes Them?

It's a fair question. If the body makes redox signaling molecules, why would I need more?

Redox signaling can decline substantially with age (reported across multiple systems), which helps explain slower healing, more inflammation, brain fog, and reduced resilience in later decades. *I summarize key research in the Resources section.*

Women over 60, in particular, often feel this decline — not only in their own bodies but also as caregivers watching loved ones suffer. Supplementing with redox is not introducing something foreign. It is **replenishing what's been lost.**

It is, quite literally, **giving the body back its native language.**

Why Redox Is Vital — Especially for Women Over 60

- **Essential for cellular communication & repair** → Redox signaling helps activate DNA repair, regulate inflammation, and coordinate immune defense.

- **Declines with age** → Natural signaling capacity can fall substantially, contributing to fatigue, chronic inflammation, and slower recovery.

- **Supports hormones & gene pathways** → Redox signaling influences insulin sensitivity, estrogen balance, serotonin, and antioxidant defenses — all crucial in later seasons of life

Objection: "It's Just Salt Water."

This is the most common — and most misguided — criticism.

Skeptics say, "It's just salt water."

But that's like saying bread is just flour, or glass is just sand. Yes, the base ingredients are water and salt — the same as your body's plasma. **After processing, it's no longer "salt water"; it's a bioactive signaling solution** created through a patented electrochemical process that reorganizes those ingredients into **a balanced mixture of reactive redox species the body uses for signaling**.

It's redox — **bioactive, native-compatible, and readily recognized** by your cells.

It's easy to misunderstand at first glance; many people are surprised by what the science actually shows once they look closer.

Divine Design — Why I Call It the God Molecule

I call redox the **God Molecule** because it is not synthetic, not a drug, not even a supplement in the usual sense. It is **native** to the human body, born inside your own cells from water and salt, powered by the energy of your mitochondria.

This is divine design.

It is the same wisdom that knows how to knit skin back together after a cut, how to grow a child in the womb, how to calm a racing heart after fear.

And redox is not unique to humans. It exists in plants, animals — all living things. It is the **universal spark of communication** that powers life itself.

Once, scientists thought redox was just "cellular noise." Now they know: **it is the language of life** — or perhaps, more truly, **the whisper of God inside the cell**.

The Science Made Simple

When redox signaling is working well:

- Cells under stress send repair signals, activating detox and healing.

- Genes switch on pathways for immune defense, inflammation control, and tissue regeneration.

- The immune system stays intelligent — targeting what needs to be destroyed, repairing what needs to be restored.

Redox molecules don't heal you.

They help your body coordinate where repair is needed.

Your body already knows how. It just needs the signal.

Redox molecules are like the cell phone signal inside your body. They don't do the work for you, but they carry the messages that let your cells talk to each other. When the signal is strong, your body knows exactly what to repair and restore. When the signal is weak or scrambled, the message doesn't get through — and healing slows down.

You don't have to understand all the science — just know that these molecules are the body's natural messengers, guiding healing where it's needed most.

The Man Who Made It Possible

For decades, scientists believed redox signaling molecules couldn't be stabilized outside the body. Then came **Dr. Gary L. Samuelson**, an atomic medical physicist who refused to give up on the puzzle.

> *"Redox signaling technology is destined to fuel the greatest advances in medical science this century."*
> — *Dr. Gary L. Samuelson, PhD, Anti-Ageing Conference London (AACL), 2013*

Through persistence and vision, Dr. Samuelson helped develop a method to stabilize **a balanced mixture of reactive redox species the body uses for signaling** and deliver them back in a usable form.

This breakthrough opened a door few thought could be opened: the ability to **replenish the signaling network** that helps keep the body alive, adaptive, and whole.

My Husband's Story: The Turning Point

Nine months into living with neuropathy pain in both arms, my husband had nearly given up hope. Then one day, he applied a small amount of redox gel to his forearm — three times, five minutes apart.

Ten minutes later, he looked at me with wide eyes.

"I feel something here," he whispered.

It wasn't just the sensation that mattered. It was the knowing. The signal had gone through. Something deep inside had reconnected.

In three weeks of drinking the liquid and applying the gel, he was pain-free. **Individual experiences vary.**

That moment changed everything for us.

Why It Matters for Women

For women, redox is more than cellular repair — it's hormonal balance, emotional resilience, and vitality.

As estrogen and progesterone decline with age, the body loses some of its natural antioxidant defenses. Mitochondria become less efficient. **Redox signaling becomes even more essential** for bone density, mood stability, memory, and energy.

For caregivers especially, redox is often the missing piece that restores the spark within. It's not about avoiding illness. It's about **keeping the inner light on** through all seasons of life.

You Are Wired for Wholeness

There is a healed version of you that already exists. **Think of it like this:** In a quantum sense, many possibilities exist at once — including the one where your body is strong, your mind is clear, your spirit is at peace.

Redox doesn't create that version. **It helps your body remember how to find it.**

It's not magic. It's not hype.

It's simply the restoration of truth at the smallest, most powerful level of life.

Final Thoughts — Return to Divine Communication

This book has never been about a prescription. It is about a reunion.

Every habit — **breath, water, food, movement, sleep, sunlight** — has been pointing to this: **restoring your original design.**

You are not broken. You are not defective.

You are a divine communication network, wired for wholeness.

Redox is the bridge between science and Spirit, the spark that lets your cells sing again.

So, remember this, luminous woman:

- You are not disconnected.

- You are being restored.

- And the light inside you is ready to shine.

Key Takeaway

Redox signaling molecules are your body's native messengers. They don't heal you — **they help coordinate the signals for repair.** Restoring redox is like turning the lights back on inside the body. For women, especially in later seasons of life, redox is a vital ally in sustaining vitality, balance, and resilience.

You don't need to be a scientist to appreciate the miracle of redox signaling. All you need to know is that your body was designed with these tiny messengers to keep repair, renewal, and protection flowing every single day. For women in their 50s, 60s, and beyond, this means hope — your body is not winding down, it is constantly working to restore you. When you honor this design with simple, life-giving habits, you awaken the God-given power already written into your cells.

Bridge to Chapter 11: The Emotional Frequency of Healing

As powerful as redox is, it is not the whole story.

Because just as your cells listen to molecules, they also listen to **frequencies.**

Love, joy, peace, gratitude — these carry resonances that shape healing as profoundly as any nutrient or molecule.

And that is where we go next.

PART THREE

Living Your Divine Design

*Where identity, emotion, and divine
design meet wholeness.*

CHAPTER 11

The Healing Power of Love, Joy, and Peace

"We were brought here with everything needed to live successfully in every area of life; however, until those truths are unfolded in one's awareness, they cannot be accessed nor applied."

—Dr. Kay Fairchild/New Life Ministries Inc.

You've now walked through the 7 Habits of Highly Healthy Women—breath, hydration, nutrition, movement, sleep, sunlight, and redox. Each one is powerful on its own, but together they form a rhythm, a symphony of healing. This is not about mastering a checklist, but about remembering your divine design—a body created to repair, renew, and thrive.

Joy, peace, and love aren't just feelings—they're biochemical signals. When the heart is at ease, the nervous system softens, hormones rebalance, and cellular communication improves. Elevated emotions shift your physiology—from redox signaling to inflammation—so your body remembers how to heal.

Long before I ever heard the term cellular health, I knew what it felt like to be in the presence of love. My shoulders dropped. My breath slowed. My mind quieted. It was as if my cells themselves were exhaling — as if they knew they were safe.

And the opposite was true as well. When conflict entered the room, my body stiffened, my jaw tightened, my thoughts scattered. No one had to tell me I was stressed — my heart rate, my stomach, and even my skin was speaking for me.

Science now confirms what our souls have always known: Emotions are not just fleeting feelings. They are biochemical events — electrical frequencies that shape our internal environment. Every thought, every feeling, every energetic exchange sends messages to our cells, turning healing on or off.

We talk about breath, hydration, nutrition, movement, sunlight, sleep, and redox molecules — but your emotional frequency is just as real, just as measurable, and just as essential to your healing as any nutrient or supplement.

How Emotions Become Biology

*"The mind and body are intimately connected,
and what we think and feel affects every cell in our body."*

— Dr. Joe Dispenza

Neuroscientist Dr. Candace Pert demonstrated that emotions aren't confined to the brain. Her research on neuropeptides revealed that emotional chemistry flows throughout the entire body, linking mind and physiology in one integrated system (Molecules of Emotion, 1997; Journal of Immunology, 1985).

When we feel joy, gratitude, or peace, our cells bathe in a chemical cascade that supports repair:

- Cortisol drops.

- Inflammation calms.

- Blood vessels open, improving circulation.

- Oxytocin and endorphins rise, enhancing immunity.

When we feel fear, resentment, or hopelessness for extended periods, the opposite occurs:

- Stress hormones flood the system.

- Digestion slows; immunity weakens.

- Inflammatory signals surge, damaging tissues over time.

Your emotions are literally instructing your cells — moment by moment — on how to behave.

Why This Especially Matters for Women

Women's bodies are exquisitely responsive to emotional frequency. Our hormonal systems are deeply tied to our relationships, environment, and sense of safety.

When a woman feels secure, loved, and valued, her body shifts into a parasympathetic state — the rest, repair, and receive mode where healing happens. Blood flows to reproductive organs, digestion improves, and cellular repair is prioritized.

But when stress is constant — whether from caregiving overload, unspoken resentment, perfectionism, or living in a state of doing rather than being — her body stays in survival mode. Cortisol remains elevated, progesterone and estrogen can become imbalanced, and cellular repair is delayed.

This is why joy, play, and meaningful connection are not luxuries for women — they are medicine.

The Measurable Power of Positive Emotion

Dr. David Hawkins, in his *Map of Consciousness*, described how emotions vibrate at measurable frequencies:

- Shame and guilt: ~20–30 Hz

- Fear: ~100 Hz

- Love: ~500 Hz

- Joy and peace: 540 Hz and above

While these numbers are symbolic, modern research has confirmed the principle: Elevated emotional states like gratitude or compassion create measurable shifts in the body.

The HeartMath Institute, for example, found that when people focus on appreciation or love for just three minutes, their immune system activity improves for hours afterward. Their heart rhythms become more coherent, their brains synchronize, and their physiology enters a state of harmony.

This is not poetic metaphor. It is biology. Love, joy, and peace literally rewire your cells for healing.

Affirmation: My joy is medicine. My peace is power. My love is life-giving.

My Story, My Mission, My Purpose

For me, this journey started, unknowingly, when my mother moved in with us. As her caregiver and health advocate, this became my personal experience and truth.

I realized that the greatest healing does not come only from prescriptions, supplements, surgeries, treatments, or even these 7 habits!

It comes when we remember who we are. When I realized that all the answers lie within, when I started to trust that still small voice, when I felt my intuition leading me to research, to learn, to get a second or third opinion, this is when I started to truly believe that we were created with the innate ability to self-heal.

There came a moment when I felt safe enough to exhale, loved enough to soften, joyful enough to laugh, and peaceful enough to rest.

This is why I share these 7 Habits of Highly Healthy Women. They are not just about food, water, or sleep. They are about restoring the sacred communication that keeps your body and your spirit whole — and my mission is to help women everywhere remember this truth for themselves.

Practices to Raise Your Emotional Frequency

Here are a few simple practices you can begin today to reorient your inner frequency toward healing:

1. Gratitude Before Screens

Before checking your phone in the morning, name three things you're thankful for — out loud. It sets your cells in a healing direction.

2. Daily Micro-Joys

Create small pockets of joy throughout the day — a favorite song, fresh flowers, sunlight on your face. I look at pictures of my grandchildren and it instantly brings joy to my heart.

3. Heart Breathing (From HeartMath)

Place your hand over your heart. Inhale for 5 seconds, exhale for 5 seconds, imagining the breath flowing in and out of your chest. While breathing, focus on a feeling of love or appreciation. (https://www.heartmath.org/articles-of-the-heart/the-math-of-heartmath/heart-focused-breathing/)

4. Release Practices

Journal your feelings, talk them through with a trusted friend, or practice gentle movement like yoga or dance to release stored tension.

The Cellular Truth

Your body listens to everything your mind says. It listens to the tone of your inner voice, the quality of your thoughts, and the frequency of your emotions.

- Love is not just a feeling — it's a physiological state that changes the chemistry of your blood.

- Joy is not just an attitude — it's a vibration that can be measured in your heart rhythm.

- Peace is not just the absence of conflict — it's the activation of your body's deepest repair systems.

When you choose love, joy, and peace, you are literally choosing to heal.

The Symphony of Habits and Emotions

Emotions don't stand apart from your body's needs — they infuse them. Breath, hydration, nutrition, movement, sleep, sunlight, and redox are the instruments. Love, joy, and peace are the music that lets them harmonize.

When you raise your emotional frequency, every single one of your habits works better. And when you practice the habits, they, in turn, lift your emotional state. This is not just lifestyle — it's resonance.

Think of your breath: When it flows with calm awareness, every inhale tells your body it is safe. Cortisol lowers, muscles soften, and even your heartbeat begins to move in rhythm with peace. Contrast that with shallow, anxious breathing, which keeps your body locked in survival.

The same is true of hydration. Hydration isn't just about volume — it carries energy. Have you ever noticed how drinking a glass of water in a moment of gratitude feels different than gulping one down in stress? Gratitude changes the way your body receives. The water becomes a messenger of calm, flowing through your bloodstream with a subtle frequency of peace.

Nutrition, too, is more than calories and nutrients. The state of your mind when you eat decides how well you absorb. A joyful, relaxed meal nourishes; a stressed, hurried one ferments poorly and leaves you depleted.

And then there is movement. When you move with joy — whether dancing in your kitchen or walking with a friend — the body not only strengthens but also clears stagnant emotions. Endorphins rise, blood circulates freely, and your cells receive the signal: She is alive, she is in flow.

Sleep, too, responds to frequency. A woman who lays her head down in a spirit of peace drifts into deep, restorative rest. But one who carries resentment, fear, or unfinished tension into bed often finds her nights restless and her mornings heavy. The frequency you carry into sleep decides how fully your body repairs itself while you dream.

Even the sunlight, the ancient healer, responds to your inner state. To stand in sunlight with gratitude is to let your body drink not only vitamin D but joy itself. The warmth on your skin seems to magnify when your heart is open — light outside harmonizing with light inside.

And finally, redox. If the habits are instruments and your emotions are music, redox is the conductor that ensures every note is heard. These molecules are the messengers, translating breath, water, food, light, sleep, and movement into clear cellular instructions. Without them, the body's communication breaks down, and the music of healing falters. With them, all becomes symphonic.

When love raises your frequency and redox molecules carry that signal, your body remembers how to heal.

The Frequency Prescription

If food is medicine for your body, emotion is medicine for your soul — and together they create the environment for your cells to thrive.

When you love daily — speaking it, feeling it, receiving it — your chemistry changes. When you laugh often, you create a ripple of nitric oxide and endorphins that relax your blood vessels and your spirit. When you let go regularly, you unburden your body as surely as you would by clearing out toxins.

Healing is not only about what you do; it is about what you feel. And every time you choose the higher frequency — love instead of resentment, joy instead of despair, peace instead of worry — you are literally choosing to heal.

Your body is always listening. Your cells are waiting for your signal.

The Invitation — Walking This Path Together

I believe you found this book for a reason. Maybe you were searching for answers no one else seemed to have. Maybe you were tired of being told your symptoms were "just part of getting older." Or maybe you've been quietly carrying the sense that you were made for more — more energy, more vitality, more joy, more life.

I wrote *The 7 Habits of Highly Healthy Women* because I know what it feels like to be in that place — to feel the tug of your own potential but not quite know how to unlock it. I also know how lonely it can feel to walk this journey without a map, or without sisters walking alongside you.

The truth is: You are not meant to do this alone. Women thrive in circles. We always have.

When women come together with the shared intention of healing, something extraordinary happens. We amplify each other's energy. We inspire courage. We remind each other that we're not broken — we're becoming.

That is why I extend this invitation to you. Not as a prescription, but as a pathway:

- To go deeper with these habits through my book and my 7 Habits in 7 Weeks campanion experience.

- To experience for yourself the profound difference redox molecules can make in restoring communication at the cellular level.

- To step into a circle of women committed to radiant health, emotional freedom, and divine connection.

This is not about doing more. It's about remembering more — who you already are, and the wholeness your body longs to return to.

A Heart-to-Heart

If I could sit with you right now — just the two of us, a pot of tea between us, no rush, no noise — I would take your hands in mine and say this:

You are not broken.

You are not behind.

You are not too late.

Your body remembers how to heal. Your spirit remembers how to shine. And every step you have taken through these habits — every glass of water, every mindful breath, every moment of rest, every laugh, every tear released — has been leading you back here: to yourself.

Sometimes the path of healing feels overwhelming, as though you have to do it all, fix it all, know it all. But what I've learned — and what I want you to hold onto — is that it's not about perfection. It's about resonance. When your choices, your emotions, and your cells are aligned with love, joy, and peace, your body naturally begins to remember its wholeness.

And you don't have to do this alone. Women have always healed best in circles, surrounded by voices that say: *I see you. I believe in you. I walk beside you.*

As we step into the final chapter together, I want you to carry this truth in your heart: Healing is not just for you, it is through you. The light you rekindle inside yourself becomes a lamp for the women who walk beside you and those who will come after you.

That is the legacy of Highly Healthy Women.

Transition Bridge

Every choice you've made to return to yourself — every breath, every glass of water, every moment of joy — is proof that healing is not something you missed out on. It is not behind you. It is within you. Right here. Right now.

And yet, what you are reclaiming is not just for you. Healing never stops at the edges of one woman's skin. It ripples outward

— into your family, your friendships, your community, and into generations yet to come.

That is why the final step of this journey is not simply about health, but about legacy. Let us walk together now into what it means to live as a Luminous, Divine Woman, carrying your light forward as a gift to the world.

CHAPTER 12

Legacy:
A Life of Health, Vitality, and Wholeness

"When a woman heals, she doesn't heal alone.
She heals her lineage, her community,
and the world around her."

—*Women's wisdom proverb (author unknown)*

If you've come this far, I want you to pause for a moment and truly honor yourself. You've walked through the **Seven Habits — Breath, Hydration, Nutrition, Movement, Sleep, Sunlight,** and **Redox**. You've explored the frequencies of love, joy, and peace. You've remembered that your body is not an obstacle but a divine design.

And now, we stand at the threshold of something greater.

This chapter is not about another habit. It is about what happens when you live these habits long enough that they become who you are. It is about your legacy.

The Quiet Ripple of Wholeness

If you have ever tossed a pebble into still water, you've seen how ripples expand far beyond the point of impact. Healing is like that. At first, it begins quietly inside of you — the deeper breaths, the glass of water, the joyful walk, the peaceful night's sleep.

But then the ripples begin.

Your family feels it when you laugh more easily. Your friends notice when your eyes shine differently. The woman at the checkout counter senses your patience. Your granddaughter remembers how you sat with her in presence, not hurry. This is legacy. It is not written only in books or bank accounts. It is written in the lives we touch through the frequency we carry.

A Circle That Extends Beyond You

Women have always healed in circles. Our ancestors gathered at fires, in kitchens, in gardens, in birthing rooms. Healing was never just an individual journey; it was communal, passed from one generation to the next.

When you embody the Seven Habits, you do more than extend your own vitality — you model what is possible for the women around you. You remind them that health is not a number on a chart but a resonance, a way of being fully alive.

And here is the beautiful truth: You don't have to be perfect to inspire others. Your very becoming — your willingness to keep showing up for yourself — is enough to awaken hope in someone else.

Redefining Legacy

We often think of legacy as something we leave behind. But legacy is also what we live right now. Every time you choose love over resentment, wholeness over fragmentation, vitality over fatigue, you are actively shaping the world your daughters, sisters, and granddaughters will inherit.

Legacy is not just what you leave.

Legacy is what you embody.

Living as a Divine Woman

A Divine Woman is not one who has done everything right. She is one who has remembered who she really is. She knows without question that she is loved, powerful, and beautiful in every sense of the word. She understands that God is living in her — as her — and therefore she has nothing to fear.

She knows how to align her body, mind, and spirit with the rhythms of nature and the signals of her own soul. She breathes deeply. She hydrates gratefully. She eats with awareness, moves with joy, rests with peace, welcomes **sunlight**, and restores her cells with the language of redox.

And because she lives this way, her very presence becomes medicine.

Her laughter lightens the room. Her calm steadies those around her. Her joy makes others believe that more is possible.

This is who you are becoming.

Passing the Flame

As we close this journey, I want you to imagine yourself years from now. Picture yourself surrounded by women you love

— daughters, nieces, friends, even strangers who have become sisters. They are watching you, listening to you, receiving from you. And what they feel most is not your words but your energy.

They feel your light.

And in that moment, they realize: *If she can live with this kind of radiance, so can I.*

That is how your legacy is born — not through striving, but through shining.

A Final Heart-to-Heart

I wrote this book not only to share information, but to share part of my story with you. As a woman in her sixties, I can look back and see moments where I didn't always show up in the best way for the people I love most. Like many women, I carried unhealed pain — and unhealed pain often spills over. Hurt people hurt people.

But here is the grace: Our mistakes are not wasted. They become teachers. They show us where we are called to grow, to take ownership, to soften, to change. In my late fifties, I began to truly awaken to this truth — that every path of healing ultimately leads back to ourselves. And when we change, the world around us changes.

This is what it means to remember your divine design: to honor the past, learn from it, and choose wholeness in the present. It is the only way forward, and it is the most powerful gift we can give to those we love.

You are not meant to walk this path alone. That is why I've created spaces where women can continue this journey together

— circles where the Seven Habits become lived practice, where redox becomes daily restoration, where your story of healing becomes part of a much greater story.

If your heart is stirring, if something within you is whispering *yes*, then I invite you to step into this circle with me. This book, the companion experience, the molecules — these are simply tools. What truly matters is the resonance we create together as women who choose to live healthy, enjoy abundant vitality, and live wholesome lives. So let this be your takeaway:

You are the legacy. You are the light. You are a Divine Woman.

The End of the Beginning

This is not the end of your journey. It is only the beginning of a new way of being — one that carries forward into every breath, every relationship, every moment still to come. May you walk forward luminous, whole, and free.

> *"You are the light of the world.*
> *A city set on a hill cannot be hidden."*
>
> *— Matthew 5:14*

As you turn the final page, remember this: Your body is not broken — it is brilliant. You are carrying within you the divine design for healing, vitality, and wholeness.

The habits you've discovered here are not complicated. They are simple, sacred rhythms woven into creation itself. When you breathe deeply, drink living water, nourish your body, move with grace, rest in peace, soak in sunlight, and honor the God molecule within — you are living your legacy.

My prayer is that you will not keep these habits to yourself. Share them with your daughters, your friends, your sisters, and the generations that follow. As you do, you'll awaken not only your own healing, but a ripple of wholeness that can transform families, communities, and beyond.

Remember who you are. And live from that truth, every single day.

Your Next Step

You've discovered the 7 Habits of Highly Healthy Women. Now it's time to begin.

1. Choose one habit today. Start small — a deep breath, a glass of water, a short walk. Small steps create lasting change.

2. Reflect daily. Ask yourself: *How did I honor my divine design today?*

3. Share your journey. Tell a friend, a daughter, or a sister about what you've learned. Healing multiplies when we walk together.

Remember who you are. You were created for healing, vitality, and wholeness.

From Remembering to Living

You've journeyed with me through these pages — from awakening to remembering — and now the invitation is to live what you've remembered.

The Seven Habits are more than ideas; they are rhythms waiting to breathe through your days. Let them weave themselves into your mornings and meals, your laughter and stillness, your prayer and your rest.

This is where real transformation takes root—not in doing more, but in remembering who you already are.

If your heart longs to go deeper, I invite you to continue the journey through *7 Habits in 7 Weeks*, a gentle companion experience designed to help you integrate each habit into daily life, week by week, breath by breath. You can find additional details and connect with me at **MiriamSpencer.com**.

And if you ever feel called to bring this message to your community or women's gatherings, I would be honored to share these teachings as part of your event or retreat.

However you choose to continue, may these habits anchor joy, renewal, and sacred remembrance in every part of your life.

With love and gratitude,
Miriam

References

AARP & National Alliance for Caregiving. (2020). *Caregiving in the United States — 2020 Report.* Washington, DC. https://doi.org/10.26419/ppi.00103.001

Afshin, A., Sur, P. J., Fay, K. A., et al. (2019). Health effects of dietary risks in 195 countries, 1990–2017. *The Lancet, 393*(10184), 1958–1972. https://doi.org/10.1016/S0140-6736(19)30041-8

Blum, H. F. (1941). *Carcinogenesis by Ultraviolet Light.* Princeton University Press.

Booth, F. W., Roberts, C. K., & Laye, M. J. (2012). Lack of exercise is a major cause of chronic diseases. *Comprehensive Physiology, 2*(2), 1143–1211. https://doi.org/10.1002/cphy.c110025

Brown, R. P., & Gerbarg, P. L. (2005). Sudarshan Kriya Yogic breathing in the treatment of stress, anxiety, and depression: Clinical applications and guidelines. *Journal of Alternative and Complementary Medicine*, 11(4), 711–717.

Centers for Disease Control and Prevention, National Center for Health Statistics. (2019). *Prescription drug use in the United States, 2015–2016* (NCHS Data Brief No. 347). https://www.cdc.gov/nchs/products/databriefs/db347.htm

Irwin, M. R. (2015). Why sleep is important for health: A psychoneuroimmunology perspective. *Annual Review of Psychology, 66*, 143–172. https://doi.org/10.1146/annurev-psych-010213-115205

Jones, D. P. (2006). Redefining oxidative stress. *Antioxidants & Redox Signaling, 8*(9–10), 1865–1879. https://doi.org/10.1089/ars.2006.8.1865

Kensler, T. W., Wakabayashi, N., & Biswal, S. (2007). Cell survival responses via the Keap1–Nrf2–ARE pathway. *Annual Review of Pharmacology and Toxicology, 47*, 89–116. https://doi.org/10.1146/annurev.pharmtox.46.120604.141046

Lew Rockwell. *Dermatology's Disastrous War Against the Sun.* (2025). https://www.lewrockwell.com/2025/06/no_author/dermatologys-disastrous-war-against-the-sun/

Lindqvist, P. G., Epstein, E., Landin-Olsson, M., et al. (2014). Avoidance of sun exposure is a risk factor for all-cause mortality. *Journal of Internal Medicine, 276*(1), 77–86. https://doi.org/10.1111/joim.12251

Midwestern Doctor. *Dermatology's Disastrous War Against the Sun.* (2025). https://www.midwesterndoctor.com/p/dermatologys-disastrous-war-against

Pedersen, B. K., & Saltin, B. (2015). Exercise as medicine. *Scandinavian Journal of Medicine & Science in Sports, 25*(S3), 1–72. https://doi.org/10.1111/sms.12581

Perrier, E. T., Armstrong, L. E., Bottin, J. H., et al. (2020). Hydration for health hypothesis: A narrative review. *European Journal of Nutrition,* 59(Suppl 1), 1–14. https://doi.org/10.1007/s00394-020-02139-5

Pinquart, M., & Sörensen, S. (2003). Differences between caregivers and noncaregivers in psychological and physical health: A meta-analysis. *Psychology and Aging,* 18(2), 250–267. https://doi.org/10.1037/0882-7974.18.2.250

Popkin, B. M., D'Anci, K. E., & Rosenberg, I. H. (2010). Water, hydration, and health. *Nutrition Reviews,* 68(8), 439–458. https://doi.org/10.1111/j.1753-4887.2010.00304.x

Russo, M. A., Santarelli, D. M., & O'Rourke, D. (2017). The physiological effects of slow breathing in the healthy human. *Breathe*, 13(4), 298–309.

Samuelson, G. L. (2010). *The Science of Healing Revealed.* Balance Publishing.

Tinetti, M. E., Fried, T. R., & Boyd, C. M. (2012). Designing health care for the most common chronic condition— multimorbidity. *JAMA*, 307(23), 2493–2494. https://doi. org/10.1001/jama.2012.5265

Walker, M. P. (2017). *Why We Sleep: Unlocking the Power of Sleep and Dreams.* New York: Scribner.

Willett, W. C., & Stampfer, M. J. (2013). Current evidence on healthy eating. *Annual Review of Public Health, 34,* 77–95. https://doi.org/10.1146/annurev-publhealth-031811-124646

Acknowledgments

I extend my deepest gratitude to **Dr. Gary L. Samuelson, Ph.D.**, atomic medical physicist, whose dedication to exploring the physics of signaling and cellular health has changed countless lives — including mine. Through his pioneering research, he unlocked the stabilization of redox signaling molecules outside the body, a discovery that opened new horizons for healing and reminded us of the incredible intelligence built into our cells.

Walking alongside Dr. Samuelson and his wife Iris, and graduating from the **Cellular Health Coaching Optimal Course in 2022**, was a transformative experience for me — one that reshaped my own health journey, deepened my teaching, and continues to inspire my coaching practice.

Dr. Samuelson's mentorship and vision remind me daily that science and spirit are not separate, but beautifully intertwined. For that, and for the gift of his work, I remain profoundly grateful.

I also wish to thank my **husband**, whose journey through pain and healing has been both my greatest challenge and my greatest teacher. His courage opened the door to redox in our lives, and his story continues to fuel my passion for helping others discover what's possible.

To my **mother**, who first brought me into the role of caregiver and advocate and ignited my awakening: your presence, your vulnerability, and your strength gave me the lens through which I now see health as sacred.

To my **family**, especially my children and grandchildren, thank you for being my daily source of joy and my reminder that every choice I make ripples forward into the generations to come. Looking at your faces is enough to lift my frequency, every single time.

To my **readers**, thank you for opening your heart to these pages. This book is not complete without you. Every time you breathe deeper, drink more water, choose joy, or embrace the light, you become part of a circle of healing women across the world.

With love, gratitude, and reverence,
Miriam

About the Author

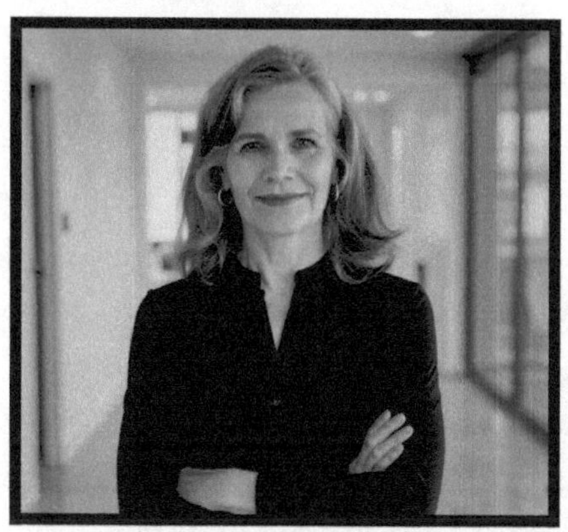

Miriam Rigal Spencer is a Certified Health and Life Coach, trained through the Health Coach Institute, and a graduate of the Cellular Health Coaching Optimal Course under Dr. Gary Samuelson, Ph.D.

Her journey into holistic health began during her years as a caregiver for her mother, where she witnessed both the limitations of conventional healthcare and the remarkable resilience of the human body. That journey deepened when her husband experienced significant healing through redox cellular communication—an experience that reshaped Miriam's understanding of how quickly the body can respond when properly supported.

Those moments awakened her to the innate intelligence within the body and inspired her to dedicate her life to helping women restore energy, vitality, and wholeness from the inside out.

Miriam is the author of *The 7 Habits of Highly Healthy Women: Discover Your Divine Design for Healing, Vitality, and Wholeness*, a transformative framework that weaves together science, spiritual wisdom, and daily lifestyle practices. Through her writing, coaching, and signature programs, she guides women—especially those in midlife and beyond—to embody habits of breath, hydration, nutrition, movement, sleep, sunlight, and redox as pathways to renewed vitality and self-trust.

Her work is grounded in a simple but powerful belief: women are not broken—they are brilliant. She writes for the woman who is ready to quiet the noise, listen to her body, and remember the divine design already within her.

Miriam is passionate about empowering women to reclaim not only their health, but also their joy, radiance, and legacy. For her, health is not merely personal—it is generational, a sacred gift passed on through families and communities.

When she is not writing or coaching, Miriam treasures time with her husband, children, and grandchildren, who remind her daily that love, laughter, and connection are among life's most powerful medicines.

To continue the journey, visit **MiriamSpencer.com** to learn more about *7 Habits in 7 Weeks*, a companion experience designed to help you live what you've discovered here.